Dental Public Health

Editors

MICHELLE M. HENSHAW
ASTHA SINGHAL

DENTAL CLINICS OF NORTH AMERICA

www.dental.theclinics.com

April 2018 • Volume 62 • Number 2

ELSEVIER

1600 John F. Kennedy Boulevard • Suite 1800 • Philadelphia, Pennsylvania, 19103-2899

http://www.dental.theclinics.com

DENTAL CLINICS OF NORTH AMERICA Volume 62, Number 2
April 2018 ISSN 0011-8532, ISBN: 978-0-323-56635-3

Editor: John Vassallo; j.vassallo@elsevier.com
Developmental Editor: Laura Fisher

Dental Clinics of North America (ISSN 0011-8532) is published quarterly by Elsevier Inc., 360 Park Avenue South, New York, NY 10010-1710. Months of issue are January, April, July, and October. Business and Editorial Offices: 1600 John F. Kennedy Boulevard, Suite 1800, Philadelphia, PA 19103-2899. Periodicals postage paid at New York, NY and additional mailing offices. Subscription prices are $294.00 per year (domestic individuals), $581.00 per year (domestic institutions), $100.00 per year (domestic students/residents), $364.00 per year (Canadian individuals), $751.00 per year (Canadian institutions), $422.00 per year (international individuals), $751.00 per year (international institutions), and $200.00 per year (international and Canadian students/residents). International air speed delivery is included in all *Clinics* subscription prices. All prices are subject to change without notice. **POSTMASTER:** Send address changes to *Dental Clinics of North America*, Elsevier Health Sciences Division, Subscription Customer Service, 3251 Riverport Lane, Maryland Heights, MO 63043. **Customer Service (orders, claims, online, change of address): Elsevier Health Sciences Division, Subscription Customer Service, 3251 Riverport Lane, Maryland Heights, MO 63043. Tel: 1-800-654-2452 (U.S. and Canada). Fax: 314-447-8029. E-mail: journalscustomer service-usa@elsevier.com (for print support); journalsonlinesupport-usa@elsevier.com (for online support).**

Reprints. For copies of 100 or more, of articles in this publication, please contact the Commercial Reprints Department, Elsevier Inc., 360 Park Avenue South, New York, NY 10010-1710. Tel.: 212-633-3874; Fax: 212-633-3820; E-mail: reprints@elsevier.com.

The Dental Clinics of North America is covered in *MEDLINE/PubMed (Index Medicus), Current Contents/Clinical Medicine, ISI/BIOMED* and *Clinahl.*

Contributors

EDITORS

MICHELLE M. HENSHAW, DDS, MPH
Associate Dean, Office of Global and Population Health, Professor, Department of Health Policy & Health Services Research, Boston University Henry M. Goldman School of Dental Medicine, Co-Director, Center for Research to Evaluate & Eliminate Dental Disparities (CREEDD), Boston, Massachusetts, USA

ASTHA SINGHAL, BDS, MPH, PhD
Assistant Professor, Department of Health Policy & Health Services Research, Boston University Henry M. Goldman School of Dental Medicine, Boston, Massachusetts, USA

AUTHORS

HOMA AMINI, DDS, MS, MPH
Clinical Professor, The Ohio State University College of Dentistry, Nationwide Children's Hospital, Columbus, Ohio, USA

AMIR AZARPAZHOOH, DDS, MSc, PhD, FRCD(C)
Faculty of Dentistry, Institute of Health Policy, Management and Evaluation, University of Toronto, Department of Dentistry, The Mount Sinai Hospital, Toronto, Ontario, Canada

PAUL S. CASAMASSIMO, DDS, MS
Professor Emeritus, The Ohio State University College of Dentistry, Nationwide Children's Hospital, Columbus, Ohio, USA

NATALIA I. CHALMERS, DDS, PhD
Diplomate, American Board of Pediatric Dentistry, Director, Analytics and Publication, DentaQuest Institute, Columbia, Maryland, USA

ELISA M. CHÁVEZ, DDS, FACD
Associate Professor, Department of Diagnostic Sciences, University of the Pacific, Arthur A. Dugoni School of Dentistry, San Francisco, California, USA

RALPH DANA, DDS, MSc, FRCD(C)
Faculty of Dentistry, University of Toronto, Toronto, Ontario, Canada

BURTON L. EDELSTEIN, DDS, MPH
Chair, Population Oral Health, Columbia University College of Dental Medicine, Professor of Dental Medicine and Health Policy and Management, Columbia University Medical Center, New York, New York, USA; Senior Fellow in Public Policy, Children's Dental Health Project, Washington, DC, USA

MARY E. FOLEY, MPH, RDH
Medicaid, Medicare, CHIP Services Dental Association, Washington, DC, USA

RAUL I. GARCIA, DMD, MMedSc, FACD
Professor and Chair, Department of Health Policy & Health Services Research,
Boston University Henry M. Goldman School of Dental Medicine, Co-Director, Center
for Research to Evaluate and Eliminate Dental Disparities (CREEDD), Boston,
Massachusetts, USA

MICHAEL GLICK, DMD
Professor and William M. Feagans Chair, The State University of New York, University at
Buffalo School of Dental Medicine, Buffalo, New York, USA

BARBARA L. GREENBERG, MSc, PhD
Professor, Chair, Department of Epidemiology and Community Health, School of Health
Sciences and Practice, New York Medical College, Valhalla, New York, USA

ERIN L. GROSS, DDS, PhD, MS
Assistant Clinical Professor, The Ohio State University College of Dentistry, Nationwide
Children's Hospital, Columbus, Ohio, USA

MATT HALL, PhD
Children's Hospital Association, Washington, DC, USA

KIMBERLY HAMMERSMITH, DDS, MPH, MS
Adjunct Assistant Clinical Professor, The Ohio State University College of Dentistry,
Nationwide Children's Hospital, Columbus, Ohio, USA

MICHELLE M. HENSHAW, DDS, MPH
Associate Dean, Office of Global and Population Health, Professor, Department of Health
Policy & Health Services Research, Boston University Henry M. Goldman School of Dental
Medicine, Co-Director, Center for Research to Evaluate and Eliminate Dental Disparities
(CREEDD), Boston, Massachusetts, USA

JEREMY A. HORST, DDS, PhD
Postdoctoral Fellow, Department of Biochemistry and Biophysics, University of California
San Francisco, San Francisco, California, USA

NIMA LAGHAPOUR, HBSc (C)
Faculty of Dentistry, University of Toronto, Toronto, Ontario, Canada

JOHN MARTIN, DDS
Chief Science Consultant, PreViser Corporation, State College, Pennsylvania, USA

SUSAN C. McKERNAN, DMD, MS, PhD
Assistant Professor, Preventive and Community Dentistry, The University of Iowa College
of Dentistry and Dental Clinics, Iowa City, Iowa, USA

PETER M. MILGROM, DDS
Professor Emeritus, Department of Oral Health Sciences, University of Washington,
Seattle, Washington, USA

SHANNON MILLS, DDS
PreViser Corporation, Concord, New Hampshire, USA

MAN WAI NG, DDS, MPH
Pediatric Dentistry, Boston Children's Hospital, Harvard School of Dental Medicine,
Boston, Massachusetts, USA

CHRISTOPHER OKUNSERI, BDS, MSc, MLS, DDPH RCS(E), FFDRCSI
Department of Clinical Services, Marquette University School of Dentistry, Milwaukee, Wisconsin, USA

HUGH SILK, MD, MPH
Professor, Department of Family Medicine and Community Health, University of Massachusetts Medical School, Medical Director, Community Healthlink, Leominster, Massachusetts, USA

ASTHA SINGHAL, BDS, MPH, PhD
Assistant Professor, Department of Health Policy & Health Services Research, Boston University Henry M. Goldman School of Dental Medicine, Boston, Massachusetts, USA

WOOSUNG SOHN, DDS, DrPH, PhD
Associate Professor, Department of Health Policy & Health Services Research, Boston University Henry M. Goldman School of Dental Medicine, Boston, Massachusetts, USA

PAUL SUBAR, DDS, EdD, FACD
Associate Professor, Director, Special Care Clinic, Hospital Dentistry Program, Arthur A. Dugoni School of Dentistry, Clinical Professor, Department of Family and Community Medicine, UCSF School of Medicine, San Francisco, California, USA

KATIE J. SUDA, PharmD, MS
Research Health Scientist, Department of Veterans Affairs, Center of Innovation for Complex Chronic Healthcare, Edward Hines, Jr. VA Hospital, Hines, Illinois, USA; Research Associate Professor, Department of Pharmacy Systems, Outcomes and Policy, University of Illinois at Chicago College of Pharmacy, Chicago, Illinois, USA

JASON M. TANZER, DMD, PhD, DHC
Section on Oral Medicine, Professor Emeritus, Department of Oral and Maxillofacial Diagnostic Sciences, University of Connecticut Health, University of Connecticut, Farmington, Connecticut, USA

CARY THURM, PhD
Children's Hospital Association, Washington, DC, USA

JANE A. WEINTRAUB, DDS, MPH
Alumni Distinguished Professor, The University of North Carolina at Chapel Hill School of Dentistry, Adjunct Professor, Health Policy and Management, Gillings School of Global Public Health, The University of North Carolina at Chapel Hill, Chapel Hill, North Carolina, USA

JOSEPH S. WISLAR, MS
Analytics and Publication, DentaQuest Institute, Columbia, Maryland, USA

ALLEN WONG, DDS, EdD, DABSCD
Professor and Director, AEGD Program, Director, Hospital Dentistry Program, University of the Pacific, Arthur A. Dugoni School of Dentistry, San Francisco, California, USA

LYNNE M. WONG, DDS
Assistant Professor, Department of Diagnostic Sciences, University of the Pacific, Arthur A. Dugoni School of Dentistry, San Francisco, California, USA

DOUGLAS A. YOUNG, DDS, EdD, MBA, MS
Professor, Department of Diagnostic Sciences, University of the Pacific, Arthur A. Dugoni School of Dentistry, San Francisco, California, USA

Contents

> Dental public health is a unique specialty of dentistry that focuses on prevention of oral diseases among populations rather than individual patients. It encompasses several complementary disciplines and greatly varies in its functions and activities. Several federal, state, local, and nonpublic entities operationalize the mission of dental public health to improve population oral health through a diverse and vibrant workforce.

> Despite improvements in the oral health status of the US population as a whole, a disproportionately higher burden of oral diseases and disorders are borne by those individuals from low-income and racial and ethnic minority groups. These differences in health status, health outcomes, or health care use between distinct socially disadvantaged and advantaged groups are well documented and known as health disparities. It is vital that members of the dental profession understand the distribution of oral health and disease across different populations and the life span and participate in developing innovative and sustainable approaches to eliminate oral health disparities.

> This article describes the evolution of nondental health providers engaging in oral health and the influences that have played a role. This discussion is followed by a review of why oral health is a natural fit for medical care, an examination of the current trends and successes in oral health education and practice in the health professions, and the need for a comprehensive approach. The article concludes by reviewing the impact these efforts are having and defining roles for each profession in the future with thoughts about what will be required to obtain these goals.

> We focus on scalable public health interventions that prevent and delay the development of caries and enhance resistance to dental caries lesions. These interventions should occur throughout the life cycle and need to be age appropriate. Mitigating disease transmission and enhancing resistance are achieved through use of various fluorides, sugar substitutes,

mechanical barriers such as pit-and-fissure sealants, and antimicrobials. A key aspect is counseling and other behavioral interventions that are designed to promote the use of disease transmission-inhibiting and tooth resistance-enhancing agents. Advocacy for public water fluoridation and sugar taxes is an appropriate dental public health activity.

Infant oral health (IOH) is a preventive service advocated by major medical and dental organizations. IOH aims to prevent early childhood caries (ECC) and impart health strategies to families for continued oral health and prevention of future caries. IOH reaches across disciplines, is low cost, and is covered by Medicaid and many private dental payers. Increasing evidence points to immediate and long-term positive oral health outcomes of reduced disease, reduction in costly care, and reduction in ECC-associated morbidities.

This article reviews considerations for oral health care associated with the most common causes of mortality and morbidity in older adults. Many of these diseases result in functional or cognitive impairments that must be considered in treatment planning to ensure appropriate, safe, and effective care for patients. Many of these considerations parallel those of adults who have lived with developmental disabilities over a lifetime, and similar principles can be applied. Systemic diseases, conditions, and their treatments can pose significant risks to oral health, which requires prevention, treatment, and advocacy for oral health care as integral to chronic disease management.

Data suggest that providers and patients have a favorable attitude toward chairside screening in the dental setting and are willing to participate in these activities. Likewise, efficacy studies indicate this strategy can effectively identify patients who are at increased risk of disease or have the presence of disease risk factors and could benefit from medical follow-up. Studies suggest it is feasible to conduct these screenings in the dental setting. Although the American Dental Association has established screening treatment codes, challenges to widespread implementation still exist, including developing a provider reimbursement strategy and the need for adequate provider training.

Opioid analgesics and antibiotics prescribed by dentists is a useful and cost-effective measure when prescribed appropriately. Common dental conditions are best managed by extracting the offending tooth, restoring the tooth with an appropriate filling material, performing root canal therapy, and/or fabricating a prosthesis for the edentulous space. Unnecessary prescription of opioid analgesics and antibiotics to treat dental pain and bacterial infection is a growing public health concern. This article highlights the state of the literature on opioid analgesic and antibiotic prescribing practices in dentistry, the impact of opioid analgesic overdose, and prevention strategies to reduce opioid analgesics and antibiotic overprescription.

This article explores trends in 3 areas of dental services use for children younger than 21 years. First, it examines the change in access to prevention, diagnostic, and treatment services over time among Medicaid-enrolled children and how access to care is affected by state-level factors. Second, it evaluates trends and health care costs associated with the treatment of oral health conditions in the operating room of pediatric hospitals. Third, it examines the trends in use of emergency departments for dental needs among children in the United States.

Innovative models of dental care delivery and coverage are emerging across oral health care systems, causing changes to treatment and benefit plans. A novel addition to these models is digital risk assessment, which offers a promising new approach that incorporates the use of a cloud-based technology platform to assess an individual patient's risk for oral disease. Risk assessment changes treatment by including risk as a modifier of treatment and as a determinant of preventive services. Benefit plans are being developed to use risk assessment to predetermine preventive benefits for patients identified at elevated risk for oral disease.

Health care costs have traditionally been provider generated, whereas payment has been split between public and private sources. There has been little pressure on health care providers to demonstrate value. The quest for value in health care financing is now widely evident as demonstrated by governmental and private sector pursuits of a 3-part aim: better health outcomes at lower cost with improved patient and population experience. Value-based approaches involve payment innovation with its attendant constraints and opportunities for innovation. This contribution posits a growing role for dental public health by exploring interfaces with these forces within the contexts of US dental care financing.

DENTAL CLINICS OF NORTH AMERICA

ISSUE OF RELATED INTEREST

Atlas of the Oral and Maxillofacial Surgery Clinics,
September 2017 (Vol. 25, No. 2)
Oral Manifestations of Systemic Diseases
Joel J. Napeñas, *Editor*
Available at: www.oralmaxsurgeryatlas.theclinics.com

Preface

The Intersection of Clinical Practice and Dental Public Health

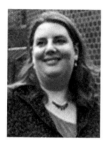 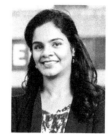

Michelle M. Henshaw, DDS, MPH   Astha Singhal, BDS, MPH, PhD
Editors

This issue of *Dental Clinics of North America* provides an overview of dental public health from the perspective that it is at the intersection of dental public health and clinical practice where significant advances will occur in improving the oral health of the US population. This is an exciting and volatile time for health care delivery in the United States, and there is intense debate about how to allocate scarce resources, whether health care is a right or a privilege, the role of the government in ensuring access to health care, and proposals for significant cuts to health care research that will have widespread implications by limiting research and slowing medical advancements. Unfortunately, dentistry has not been at the forefront of these discussions, and it is challenging to predict the impact on the profession.

What is known, however, is that dentistry and the dental care delivery system will be facing significant challenges. National data clearly demonstrate that the changing US demographics, with increases in older, ethnic minority, and poor populations, will lead to a population with increased levels of oral diseases and dental need. The existing dental care delivery system works well for the populations that can access it; however, these populations tend to be those with the lowest risk of oral disease, and the individuals who need dental care the most are the least likely to have affordable access to dental care. While some progress has been made, the oral health disparities described in the Surgeon General's Report on Oral Health are still present, and much more work needs to be done to ensure that optimal oral health is experienced by all.

Prevention is the cornerstone of dental public health, and several advances have been made in preventive therapies over the past decades. While certain preventive strategies have proven to be effective time and again, such as community water fluoridation, newer strategies such as silver diamine fluoride, atraumatic restorative therapy, and other antibacterials have now been shown to be effective complementary preventive agents. Moreover, emerging models of alternative dental providers, such as dental therapists, show promising potential in mitigating some of the barriers to dental access. This is

Dent Clin N Am 62 (2018) xi–xiii
https://doi.org/10.1016/j.cden.2018.01.001
0011-8532/18/© 2018 Published by Elsevier Inc.

especially true among the vulnerable populations, such as the low-income, publicly insured, and rural residents in states that authorize alternative dental providers. In addition, nondental providers are playing a significant role in expanding access to populations that do not regularly seek dental care but frequently connect with the medical care system, such as very young children and the geriatric population. Where, on one hand nondental providers are expanding dental access, on the other, dental providers are uniquely placed to provide systemic disease screening and can be the point of first diagnoses of systemic diseases for their patients. As the dental profession strives for greater integration with the broader health care system, it needs to be cognizant of the ongoing and emerging public health issues, such as the prescription opioid abuse epidemic.

Evolving technological changes also are shaping the profession. For example, the emergence of electronic medical and dental records and claims and billing data provides new opportunities for monitoring the quality and effectiveness of dental services provided in practice. This will allow the federal and state governments, third-party payers, and other stakeholders to develop and implement more evidence-based practice guidelines. It also may allow for different reimbursement schemes where dentists' reimbursement is based on the quality of care they provide to their patients as opposed to the number of treatments performed. This has the potential to ensure that limited public and private funds are used most effectively.

All of the aforementioned factors will likely lead to changes in the organization, delivery, and financing of dental care, and dental public health will become increasingly important and relevant to the clinical practice of dentistry. As a specialty, dental public health professionals provide expertise in understanding the distribution and trends of dental disease, planning, implementation, and evaluation of new, cost-effective models of population-based preventive and therapeutic dental care for underserved populations and public policy. These are all vital skills that must be utilized so that the dental profession takes a proactive approach to shaping the future of the profession as opposed to a more reactive approach. However, the dental profession can't do this alone. In order to develop the best solutions to the challenges facing the profession, it is clear that the profession of dentistry and the discipline of dental public health must actively engage with national, state, and local government, other health professionals, professional associations, educators, researchers, private industry, community organizations, and consumers. It is through these interactions that we will most effectively address the new challenge of the increasing rates of oropharyngeal cancer In white men, largely related to human papillomavirus, ensure access to preventive and therapeutic services to the most vulnerable populations, and develop the most cost-effective models to address the needs of the rapidly growing geriatric population, and most importantly, ensure optimal oral health for all segments of the US population.

Michelle M. Henshaw, DDS, MPH
Office of Global & Population Health
Boston University
Henry M. Goldman School of Dental Medicine
560 Harrison Avenue, 3rd Floor
Boston, MA 02118, USA

Astha Singhal, BDS, MPH, PhD
Department of Health Policy and
Health Services Research
Boston University

Henry M. Goldman School of Dental Medicine
560 Harrison Avenue #342
Boston, MA 02118, USA

E-mail addresses:
mhenshaw@bu.edu (M.M. Henshaw)
asinghal@bu.edu (A. Singhal)

Dental Public Health Practice, Infrastructure, and Workforce in the United States

Astha Singhal, BDS, MPH, PhD[a],*, Susan C. McKernan, DMD, MS, PhD[b],
Woosung Sohn, DDS, DrPH, PhD[a]

KEYWORDS

- Dental public health • Access to dental care • Dental workforce
- Alternative dental providers

KEY POINTS

- Dental public health is one of the nine specialties of dentistry that are recognized by the American Dental Association.
- Dental public health focuses on prevention of oral diseases and improving oral health of vulnerable populations.
- The infrastructure comprises a wide range of federal, state, local, and private organizations that employ dental public health workforce to operationalize the mission of dental public health, that is, to improve population oral health.

INTRODUCTION

The dental profession is primarily responsible for the oral health of patients, and dental public health evolved from it to address oral health at a population level with a strong emphasis on prevention of oral diseases and ensuring provision of adequate preventive and treatment services among vulnerable groups. Dental public health is a unique discipline that is formed by a marriage of multiple broad fields that include dentistry and public health. Hence the definition, scope, and infrastructure included under dental public health are broad and varied.

DEFINITION OF DENTAL PUBLIC HEALTH

The American Dental Association (ADA) defines the vision of dentistry as "Improved health quality of life for all through optimal oral health" and its mission is to "protect

[a] Department of Health Policy & Health Services Research, Boston University Henry M. Goldman School of Dental Medicine, 560 Harrison Avenue, Boston, MA 02118, USA; [b] Preventive and Community Dentistry, University of Iowa College of Dentistry and Dental Clinics, 801 Newton Road, Iowa City, IA 52242, USA
* Corresponding author. 560 Harrison Avenue, 3rd Floor Suite #342, Boston, MA 02118.
E-mail address: asinghal@bu.edu

Dent Clin N Am 62 (2018) 155–175
https://doi.org/10.1016/j.cden.2017.11.001
0011-8532/18/© 2018 Elsevier Inc. All rights reserved.

dental.theclinics.com

and preserve the oral health of public." Dental public health is an integral part of this mission and it is one of the nine specialties of dentistry. It was established and recognized by the ADA as a dental specialty in 1950.[1,2]

Dental public health is also a field of study within the broader discipline of public health. A widely accepted traditional definition of public health is "the science and art of preventing disease, prolonging life and promoting human health through organized efforts and informed choices of society, organizations, public and private, communities and individuals."[3] The Institute of Medicine (IOM) defines public health as "activities that society undertakes to assure the conditions in which people can be healthy. This includes organized community efforts to prevent, identify, and counter threats to the health of the public." IOM also identified the broad mission of public health as to "fulfill society's interest in assuring conditions in which people can be healthy."[4]

The professional certifying board in the field of dental public health, American Board of Dental Public Health (ABDPH) and its parent host organization, the American Association of Public Health Dentistry (AAPHD), have defined dental public health as "the science and art of preventing and controlling dental diseases and promoting dental health through organized community efforts. It is that form of dental practice that serves the community as a patient rather than the individual. It is concerned with the dental education of the public, with applied dental research, and with the administration of group dental care programs as well as the prevention and control of dental diseases on a community basis."[5]

SCOPE AND PRACTICE OF DENTAL PUBLIC HEALTH

Dental public health distinguishes itself from other disciplines of dentistry in its pursuit and practice to achieve the goal of oral health. Unlike dental practitioners and all other dental specialties that focus on individual patients' oral health, dental public health focuses on group of individuals or populations.

The conventional view of dental public health limits its scope to disease prevention (ie, fluorides, sealants, and oral health education) and mainly providing oral health care services to the most vulnerable populations. Although these are its major concerns, dental public health also has a much wider scope and practice. Reflecting on the mission of public health by the IOM, the scope and mission of dental public health is to prevent oral disease and promote oral health and general health and well-being, by ensuring the conditions in which people can achieve highest level of oral health.

The World Health Organization defines oral health as follows[6]:

Oral health is essential to general health and quality of life. It is a state of being free from mouth and facial pain, oral and throat cancer, oral infection and sores, periodontal (gum) disease, tooth decay, tooth loss, and other diseases and disorders that limit an individual's capacity in biting, chewing, smiling, speaking, and psychosocial wellbeing.

Similarly, the World Dental Federation defines oral health as follows[7]:

Oral health is multi-faceted and includes the ability to speak, smile, smell, taste, touch, chew, swallow and convey a range of emotions through facial expressions with confidence and without pain, discomfort and disease of the craniofacial complex. Further attributes of oral health include the following:

- It is a fundamental component of health and physical and mental well-being. It exists along a continuum influenced by the values and attitudes of individuals and communities;

- It reflects the physiologic, social and psychological attributes that are essential to the quality of life;
- It is influenced by the individual's changing experiences, perceptions, expectations and ability to adapt to circumstances

Clearly, the scope of dental public health to improve oral health should embrace not only physical but also psychosocial health and well-being, including social functions, connections, and interactions with one another. The field also expands its practice to improving the dental care delivery system and effective and efficient payment systems for dental services to ensure an effective, economical, and sustainable dental care delivery system for the public. This wide and complex scope of dental public health practice increasingly demands a wide range of advanced knowledge, skills, and experience in dental, behavioral, public health, education, social, and political sciences from dental public health workers.

SPECIALTY RECOGNITION

Dental public health is one of the nine dental specialties recognized by the ADA. ADA recognizes DPH as "unique among the specialties in that it is not primarily a clinical specialty; it is a specialty whose practitioners focus on dental and oral health issues in communities and populations rather than individual patients" and "part of dentistry providing leadership and expertise in population-based dentistry, oral health surveillance, policy development, community-based disease prevention and health promotion, and the maintenance of the dental safety net".

Accordingly, dental public health practice requires comprehension of an additional body of knowledge and a set of skills beyond those obtained in a predoctoral dental education. To be certified as specialists in dental public health, educational and training requirements are specified by the Commission on Dental Accreditation (CODA).[5]

As of December 31, 2017, there were 228 active ABDPH-certified diplomates.[8] Considering that there were 196,441 professionally active dentists in the United States in 2016,[9] dental public health specialists comprise less than 0.08% of all active dentists, thus making dental public health one of the smallest dental specialties. However, there were 732 dentists who identified their work as being in the area of public health dentistry, comprising about 0.37% of all active dentists in 2016.[9] This demonstrates that even though formally board-certified dental public health specialists are few, other dental professionals' activities contribute to the work of dental public health.

COMPETENCIES IN DENTAL PUBLIC HEALTH

Specific dental public health expertise is required to ensure oral health and groups of people, or populations of concern. Advanced education and training in such areas as epidemiology, biostatistics, policy, management, administration, and research provide tools to help a population achieve better oral health. There are certain foundational knowledge, practical understanding and skills, and professional values that a dental public health professional must possess to be effective in the practice of public health. These competencies provide guidance for dental public health specialists' education and qualifications and benchmarks for specialty education and training.

The early attempts to establish dental public health competencies identified 165 competency objectives under the following four broad categories (1988)[10]: (1) health policy and program management, (2) research methods in dental public health, (3) oral health promotion and disease prevention, and (4) oral health services and delivery.

In 1998, a total of 10 competencies were identified (**Table 1**), which emphasized practical skills in addition to knowledge that a specialist trained in dental public health is

Table 1
Dental public health competencies, 1998 and 2016

1998 Competences	New Competencies
1. Plan oral health programs for populations	
2. Select interventions and strategies for the prevention and control of oral diseases and promotion of oral health	
3. Develop resources, implement and manage oral health programs for populations	1. Manage oral health programs for population health
4. Incorporate ethical standards in oral health programs and activities	3. Demonstrate ethical decision-making in the practice of dental public health
5. Evaluate and monitor dental care delivery systems	2. Evaluate systems of care that impact oral health
6. Design and understand the use of surveillance systems to monitor oral health	4. Design surveillance systems to measure oral health status and its determinants
7. Communicate and collaborate with groups and individuals on oral health issues	5. Communicate on oral and public health issues 6. Lead collaborations on oral and public health issues
8. Advocate for, implement, and evaluate publish health policy, legislation, and regulations to protect and promote the public's oral health	7. Advocate for public health policy, legislation, and regulations to protect and promote the public's oral health, and overall health
9. Critique and synthesize scientific literature	8. Critically appraise evidence to address oral health issues for individuals and populations
10. Design and conduct population-based studies to answer oral and public health questions	9. Conduct research to address oral and public health problems
	10. Integrate the social determinants of health into dental public health practice

From Altman D, Mascarenhas AK. New competencies for the 21st century dental public health specialist. J Public Health Dent 2016;76:S21; with permission.

expected to master.[11] Since then, society and individual lives have undergone significant changes: arrival of the digital age, changes in demographics and disease patterns, economic instability, and changes in social trends, to name a few. There are also widening gaps between the rich and the poor in health and access to health care, changes in health care delivery system and its finance, and advancement of science and new discoveries. All of these changes impose new challenges to dental public health specialists in the practice of improving population oral health.[12] In 2016, the ABDPH, in partnership with the AAPHD and others, updated competencies for the dental public health specialist as listed in **Table 1**.[13] The new competencies are expected to provide better guidelines for the expertise of dental public health specialists in the twenty-first century.

PREVENTION: CORNERSTONE OF DENTAL PUBLIC HEALTH

Although the new competencies do not include specifically the word "prevention," it is the cornerstone of dental public health. The field has had exemplary achievements in primary prevention of oral disease at the population level. The discovery of fluorides for caries prevention and wide dissemination of community water fluoridation are epic examples of dental public health's focus and success in primary prevention at the population level. With the introduction of fluorides, most populations in the United States no longer experience severe and rampant tooth decay, pain and swelling, or early loss of their teeth - common features of life in the first half of the twentieth century. Consequently, community water fluoridation for caries prevention was recognized by the Centers for Disease Control and Prevention (CDC) as 1 of 10 great achievements in prevention during the twentieth century.[14] Community water fluoridation specifically demonstrates dental public health's strategies to prevent oral disease and promote oral health at population level rather than individual level, by ensuring "conditions in which people can be healthy."[4] Ubiquitous use of fluoridated toothpaste, school-based dental sealants, and fluoride varnish programs also exemplify primary prevention strategies of dental public health.

Poor oral health and oral diseases, such as dental caries, periodontal disease, and oral cancer, develop through a multifactorial process that includes biologic, behavioral, psychosocial, and socioenvironmental determinants.[15] Hence, preventing oral disease from developing also requires multilevel complex solutions. Dental public health professionals conceptualize this complexity and develop preventive approaches that target factors at various levels of risk and stages of disease, drawing on primary, and to a lesser extent, secondary and tertiary prevention.

Public health does not only affect population health, but it is an essential component of social justice.[16] The World Health Organization Constitution enshrines "...the highest attainable standard of health as a fundamental right of every human being."[17] Dental public health also aims to ensure equitable and just access to resources and living conditions to enable optimal oral and overall health and benefit all sections of the society. An example is community water fluoridation, a primary prevention approach that benefits all individuals who drink fluoridated water through community water supply regardless of their income level, employment, age, gender, and race/ethnicity. This exhibits dental public health's commitment to the mission of public health by ensuring that the environment in which all people lead their lives promotes health and social justice; everyone is entitled to the conditions that can maintain health.[16,17] Because dental public health plays an integral role in carrying out this societal function, it often includes advocating for and providing services for vulnerable and disadvantaged population, such as children, the elderly, the low income, the developmentally disabled, uninsured or underinsured, and racial/ethnic and cultural minorities.

CORE FUNCTIONS OF (DENTAL) PUBLIC HEALTH

Public health comprises a wide variety of functions and services, which are classified into 10 essential services that form a framework (**Fig. 1**). These 10 essential services are broadly grouped into three core public health functions (1) assessment, (2) policy development, and (3) assurance. **Fig. 1** shows how the 10 essential services align within the three core functions of public health. These core functions were first outlined in the 1988 IOM report "The Future of Public Health."[4]

Assessment

The core function of assessment includes collection, assembly, analyses, and distribution of information on the community's health. It includes the following two essential public health services:

1. Monitor health status to identify community health problems: This includes accurate and periodic assessment of the community's health status to identify health

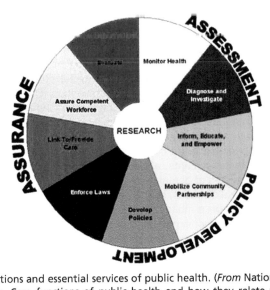

Fig. 1. Core functions and essential services of public health. (*From* National Center for Environmental Health. Core functions of public health and how they relate to the 10 essential services. Available at: https://www.cdc.gov/nceh/ehs/ephli/core_ess.htm. Accessed July 23, 2017.)

risks, disparities, and barriers and resources to address them. Examples of this type of activity are surveillance and maintaining health registries.

2. Diagnose and investigate health problems and health hazards in the community: Using regularly collected information to identify and investigate threats to community health and plan a response to address such threats. Examples of this activity are epidemiologic investigations of disease outbreaks.

Policy Development

Like the name suggests, this core function involves the development of comprehensive policies based on scientific knowledge and decision making. It includes the following essential public health functions:

3. Inform, educate, and empower people about health issues: This essential service relates to how well-informed the community is about health issues facing them. It involves such activities as health education and promotion programs and making health educational resources available and accessible.
4. Mobilize community partnerships to identify and solve health problems: This service reflects how are community members engage to solve health problems that arise. It involves such activities as community engagement, coalition building, and identifying and working with stakeholders to address threats to community health.
5. Develop policies and plans that support individual and community health efforts: This relates to how public and private policies promote community health. Activities include appropriate resource allocation to ensure optimal health and systematic health planning and emergency preparedness at all levels of the population.

Assurance

Assurance refers to making sure that all needed health services are available. It focuses on maintaining a competent capacity of public and personal health services. It includes the following essential public health services:

6. Enforce laws and regulations that protect health and ensure safety: This refers to enforcing existing laws in a competent, fair, and effective manner. This includes reviewing and evaluating existing laws, educating the community about them, and also advocating for new regulations to promote health.
7. Ensure a competent public health and personal health care workforce: Making sure that the health workforce is competent and up to date with new developments is included under this essential service. Examples of activities include cultural competency training and regular review of public health competencies and credentialing.
8. Link people to needed personal health services and ensure the provision of health care when otherwise unavailable: Identifying population groups that are facing barriers to care and ensuring an effective entry to health care system, to facilitate ongoing care are the foundation of this essential service. Examples of activities include enabling services, such as providing transportation, day care, or care coordination to facilitate health care access.
9. Evaluate effectiveness, accessibility, and quality of personal and population-based health services: Ongoing evaluation of personal and population health services must be conducted to improve quality and performance of these services. An example is examination of use of care to identify their effectiveness.
10. Research for new insights and innovative solutions to environmental health problems: This involves ensuring that new ways to achieve better health for the community are being discovered and used. It includes identifying and monitoring innovative methods to advance public health. Examples include epidemiologic, health policy, and health systems research.

INFRASTRUCTURE OF DENTAL PUBLIC HEALTH

Several public and private organizations at federal, state, and local levels perform activities that fall under several core functions and provide essential services as described previously. These organizations play a unique role in ensuring optimal health of the communities. Many of these organizations are described next.

United States Department of Health and Human Services

The US Department of Health and Human Services (HHS) is the principal federal agency that administers public health programs in the United States. The HHS has a stated priority of protecting the health of all Americans and providing essential human services, especially for those least able to help themselves. The President's budget for the HHS for fiscal year (FY) 2017 was $1145 billion and the HHS has approximately 79,400 full-time equivalent employees of personnel.[18]

Unite States Public Health Services

The US Public Health Service is one of the seven uniformed services in the nation and is comprised of more than 6,000 Commissioned Corps Officers and 50,000 Civil Service health professionals who serve in the HHS and other federal agencies. The Surgeon General heads this uniformed commissioned corps. The Chief Dental Officer is appointed by the US Surgeon General and is responsible for providing leadership, coordination, and professional growth of the dental personnel in the Public Health Service. In 2017, there were more than 600 Commissioned Corps and Civil service dentists.[19]

Indian Health Services

The Indian Health Service is the primary health care provider and health care advocate for American Indian and Alaska Native communities. The Indian Health Service serves a population of 2.2 million American Indians and Alaska Natives across 36 states belonging to 567 federally recognized tribes.[20] The Indian Health Service has been actively involved in the development of programs to address the oral health needs of rural Alaska Natives who have substantial difficulty in accessing oral health services.[21]

Centers for Disease Control and Prevention

The mission of the CDC is to promote health and quality of life by preventing and controlling disease, injury, and disability. For FY 2017, the President's budget request for the CDC was $6.98 billion.[22] The Division of Oral Health (DOH) is 1 of 10 divisions within the National Center for Chronic Disease Prevention and Health Promotion, with a budget of $14.4 million in FY 2010.[23] The DOH helps states, territories, and other countries collect oral health data, apply new methods for oral health surveillance, monitor the status of community water fluoridation, and train state and local fluoridation engineers and state program leaders on fluoridation. The DOH also promotes and provides technical assistance on school-based and school-linked dental sealant programs, investigates outbreaks of infectious diseases in clinical dental settings, and provides infection control information for dental personnel and serves as a resource within CDC on oral health. In addition, CDC also hosts a residency program in dental public health. The goals of DOH are

- To prevent and control dental caries (tooth decay) across the life stages
- To prevent and control periodontal (gum) disease
- To prevent and control oral and pharyngeal (throat) cancers and their risk factors
- To eliminate disparities in oral health
- To promote prevention of disease transmission in dental health care settings
- To increase state oral health program capacity and effectiveness

National Center for Health Statistics

The National Center for Health Statistics is the nation's principal agency for providing health statistics and it is a part of the CDC. This information is used to develop policies and programs to improve health. Oral health-related activities at the National Center for Health Statistics are primarily concentrated in the Division of Health and Nutrition Examination Surveys, which is responsible for planning, implementing, conducting, and evaluating examination and nutrition surveys at National Center for Health Statistics.

Office of Disease Prevention and Health Promotion and Healthy People 2020

Healthy People 2020 is a set of health objectives for the nation to be achieved by 2020 and administered by the Office of Disease Prevention and Health Promotion. Oral health is 1 of 42 priority areas, with 17 objectives and many subobjectives and a target of 10% improvement over the decade from baseline. The oral health objectives are for preventing and controlling oral and craniofacial diseases, conditions, and injuries, and improving access to related services. Healthy People 2020 is available at www.healthypeople.gov.[24]

National Institutes of Health

The National Institutes of Health is the primary federal agency conducting and supporting medical research, with an annual budget of more than $32 billion.[25] The discoveries from these institutes have prevented diseases and improved the quality of people's lives. This 100-year HHS agency achieves this by awarding competitive grants to researchers in its own laboratories, universities, medical and dental schools, and other research institutions. The National Institutes of Health is made up of 27 different components, called institutes and centers, with specific research agendas, such as the National Cancer Institute, National Institute of Mental Health, and others.

National Institute of Dental and Craniofacial Research (NIDCR) is one of the National Institutes of Health Institutes. The organizational mission is accomplished by:

- Performing and supporting basic and clinical research
- Conducting and funding research training and career development programs to ensure an adequate number of talented, well-prepared, and diverse investigators
- Coordinating and assisting relevant research and research-related activities among all sectors of the research community
- Promoting the timely transfer of knowledge gained from research and implications for health to the public, health professionals, researchers, and policy makers

The NIDCR plans, develops, and manages basic, translational, and clinical research supported by grants, cooperative agreements, and contracts in dental, oral, and craniofacial health and disease. Some of the areas into which research is being done include infectious diseases, health disparities, behavioral and social aspects of health and disease, temporomandibular joint dysfunction, developmental biology and mammalian genetics, AIDS and oral manifestations of immunosuppression, biomaterials, and tissue engineering and regenerative medicine. The NIDCR annual budget is about $400 million, 75% of which is distributed to grantees at universities, dental schools, and medical schools in the United States.[26]

Health Resources and Services Administration

The primary purpose of the Health Resources and Services Administration (HRSA) is to improve access to health care services for people who are uninsured, isolated, or medically vulnerable.[27] HRSA grantees provide health care in all states to uninsured people; people living with human immunodeficiency virus (HIV)/AIDS; and pregnant women, mothers, and children. HRSA activities are managed centrally and through the 10 public health service regions, some of which have dental consultants with mostly nondental responsibilities. The bureaus most active in oral health are HIV/AIDS, Maternal and Child Health, Primary Health Care, and Health Professions. In addition, HRSA developed the Integrating Oral Health and Primary Care Practice initiative that seeks to improve knowledge and skills of primary care clinicians and promote interprofessional collaborations.[28] In 2013, HRSA awarded funds to pilot five oral health competencies in three health centers to the National Network for Oral Health Access.[28]

The HIV/AIDS Bureau provides clinical care and support for uninsured and underinsured individuals and families of individuals with HIV/AIDS. All parts of the Ryan White HIV/AIDS Program support the provision of oral health services for the recipients. Specifically, the Dental Reimbursement Program and the Community-Based Dental Partnership Program provide funds for dental services and education and training of oral health providers.[29] In 2010, almost $80 million was spent on oral health within all Ryan White HIV/AIDS Program parts and more than 141,000 clients received oral health care services.[30]

The Maternal and Child Health Bureau is responsible for ensuring that necessary services are made available to American mothers and children. Programs coordinated by the Maternal and Child Health Bureau, which include oral health, have as their objective to support the development and implementation of comprehensive, cultur-ally competent, coordinated systems of care for children who have or are at risk for chronic, physical, developmental, behavioral, or emotional conditions, and who also require health and related services of a type or amount beyond that required by chil-dren generally.[28] Within the Bureau, the National Maternal and Child Oral Health Resource Center strengthens state and community oral health programs that increase access to quality oral health care for all maternal and child health populations through knowledge building, program development, and information sharing.[28]

Several other programs within HRSA address oral health, including the Office of Planning, Analyses and Evaluation; Bureau of Health Workforce; Bureau of Primary Health Care; and Office of Rural Health Policy.

National Health Service Corps

This HRSA program provides incentives to health professionals to work in commu-nities that would otherwise be without health care. Some of the strategies adopted by the National Health Service Corps are forming partnerships with communities and organizations, student loan repayment, and recruiting culturally competent clinicians.[31] The National Health Service Corps program has field strength of more than 1000 dentists and dental hygienists as of October 2010.[32] Currently, the National Health Service Corps uses loan repayment as the main incentive to attract profes-sionals to work with underserved populations. Fully trained and licensed dentists and dental hygienists may receive an initial, tax-free loan repayment award up to $60,000 for 2 years of service. Continued service provides the opportunity to pay off all dental profession student loans.[32]

Centers for Medicare and Medicaid Services

The Centers for Medicare and Medicaid Services (CMS) is the federal agency respon-sible for administering the Medicare, Medicaid, the Children's Health Insurance Pro-gram (CHIP), and the Health Insurance Marketplace. Medicaid is the federal- and state-funded program that offers benefits to eligible low-income and needy individuals and families. States are required to provide dental benefits to children covered by Medicaid and CHIP but dental benefits are optional for adults covered by Medicaid.[33] Children enrolled in Medicaid receive dental coverage under the Early and Periodic Screening, Diagnostic and Treatment program. CMS has made important progress in improving access to dental care among children. For example, from 2007 to 2011, almost half of all states (24) achieved at least a 10 percentage point increase in the proportion of children enrolled in Medicaid and CHIP that received a preventive dental service during the reporting year.[34]

The dental public health workforce is often intimately involved on the national, state, and local level, helping to improve these CMS programs and to provide access to these resources for vulnerable populations. There are two public health dentists who work in the CMS. CMS launched an Oral Health Initiative in April 2010, with a national goal to have at least 52% of enrolled children ages 1 to 20 receive a preven-tive dental service in federal FY 2015. Each state has its own federal FY 2011 baseline and federal FY 2015 goal, with interim yearly improvement goals of 2 percentage points. Between federal FY 2011 (baseline) and federal FY 2012, a total of 15 states achieved at least 2 percentage point improvement in use of preventive dental services.[35]

Medicare is the federal government–sponsored and –funded health insurance pro-gram that covers people who are older than 65 years and people less than 65 years who have certain disabilities or end-stage renal disease. It is administered in Parts

A, B, C, and D for hospital care, outpatient visits, and prescription drugs. Dental benefits are not routinely covered under Medicare, except under certain conditions, such as oral cancer.[36]

Agency for Healthcare Research and Quality

The agency for Healthcare Research and Quality (AHRQ) is a federal agency that invests in research on the nation's health delivery system that goes beyond the "what" of health care to understand the "how" to make health care safer and of better quality. It also helps by creating materials and tools to teach and train health care systems and providers to put research into practice, and generating measures and data used by providers and policymakers.[37]

The agency collects and provides data for research and administrative purposes, some of which focus on oral health. For example, the Dental Plan Survey asks patients to report on their experiences with care and services from a dental plan, the dentists, and their staff.[38] Another major source of secondary data on dental care use in the United States is the Medical Expenditure Panel Survey (MEPS), conducted by AHRQ. The MEPS is a set of large-scale surveys of families and individuals, their medical providers, and employers across the United States. MEPS is the most complete source of national data on the cost and use of health care and health insurance coverage.[39]

Food and Drug Administration

The Food and Drug Administration is responsible for protecting the public's health by ensuring the safety, efficacy, and security of human and veterinary drugs, biologic products, medical devices, the nation's food supply, cosmetics, and products that emit radiation.

State Dental Public Health Infrastructure and Oral Health Programs

Each state's department of health is important for improving the oral health of the populations they serve. Most states have a dental director who coordinates efforts and helps ensure that necessary programs and services are provided. These may include, but are not limited to, programs for the following[40]:

- Access to oral health services and workforce studies
- Early childhood caries (formerly baby bottle tooth decay)
- Fluoridation advocacy
- School fluoride mouth rinse and dental sealants
- Fluoride supplements and fluoride varnish
- Mouth-guard and injury prevention
- Clinical services and infection control
- Dental screening, needs assessment, and oral health surveys
- Oral health education and promotion
- Smoke and spit tobacco cessation
- Water fluoridation monitoring and private well fluoride testing
- Prevent abuse and neglect through dental awareness

State dental directors may be full-time or part-time. There is considerable variation in the professional training and academic qualification of these directors. As of 2014, a total of 46 states had a full-time state dental director position.[41] Of the 46 filled positions 24 were managed by a dental public health professional. The budget for dental activities in different states in 2014 to 2015 ranged from $183,377 to $5,878,386.[41] In 2014 to 2015, 12% of the states spent less than $500,000 on dental programs.[41]

Local Health Department Infrastructure and Oral Health Programs

The local health departments (LHDs) in the cities, towns, and counties of the United States are the building block of a functioning public health infrastructure. They are defined as an administrative or service unit of local or state government concerned with health, and carrying some responsibility for the health of a jurisdiction smaller than the state.[42] The LHDs are meant to understand the unique health problems facing their communities and develop programs and policies to meet these needs. They are guided by a set of regulations that ensure they offer services to improve the health of their jurisdiction. In 2016, there were 2,533 LHDs in the United States.[43] Rhode Island and Hawaii do not have any substate units, hence no LHDs. All of these health departments are unique in their size, activities, jurisdiction, and infrastructure.[43] In the 2016 National Profile of Local Health Department Report, about 50% of LHDs assessed gaps in access to dental care, 32% to 37% of LHDs implemented strategies to target and increase accessibility of existing services, and 24% of LHDs addressed gaps through direct provision of dental services.[43]

Dental Safety Net

The dental safety net comprises the facilities, providers, and payment programs that support the provision of dental care for the underserved populations.[44] This is distinct from the broader dental care delivery system, which does not have a specific focus on care provision to the underserved populations. Although several sociodemographic factors are associated with access to dental care, cost is one of the biggest barriers to accessing dental care.[45] Hence, an underserved population is most often identified based on the household income, in addition to age, health status, geographic location, and language.

The dental safety net is heterogeneous and varies considerably in availability, comprehensiveness, continuity, and quality of care.[44] The Federally Qualified Health Centers (FQHCs) and other community health centers form a significant part of the safety net. These health centers serve low-income residents, migrants, homeless, public housing residents, and racial-ethnic minorities. Health centers serve as a medical home for more than 24 million people nationally. More than 70% of FQHC patients have incomes at or below poverty level, 47% have Medicaid, 28% are uninsured, and about 50% reside in rural parts of the country.[46]

Other than the health centers, dental schools, dental hygiene programs, and mobile dental programs, private practices that serve a high proportion of underserved patients and other volunteer free care programs also form essential components of the safety net. Lastly, hospital emergency rooms serve as a part of the safety net, often as a last resort for patients to seek care.

PROFESSIONAL ORGANIZATIONS
American Public Health Association, Oral Health Section

The American Public Health Association (APHA), founded in 1872, is the oldest and largest public health association in the world. It is also the Secretariat for the World Federation of Public Health Associations and publishes the *American Journal of Public Health*. Because APHA is a multidisciplinary public health association, it provides its dental public health members with a forum to obtain support for oral health programs and initiatives from nondental public health leaders and decision makers. The members of the Oral Health Section in APHA promote oral health issues that are in the public's interest to a large multidisciplinary audience.[47]

American Association of Public Health Dentistry

The AAPHD began in 1937 and strives to improve oral health through promotion of effective efforts in disease prevention, health promotion, and service delivery; education of the public, health professionals, and decision makers regarding the importance of oral health to total well-being; and expansion of the knowledge base of dental public health and fostering competency in its practice.[48]

The AAPHD started as a group of state dental directors with restricted membership. Since then the membership criteria has been broadened to include any one working to improve oral health.[48] The AAPHD is the sponsor of the American Board of Public Health, publishes the *Journal of Public Health Dentistry*, and is a cosponsor of the yearly National Oral Health Conference with the Association of State and Territorial Dental Directors (ASTDD).

American Board of Dental Public Health

The ABDPH is a not-for-profit organization incorporated in 1950, and is the national examining and certifying agency for the specialty of dental public health. The Board was organized in accordance with the Requirements for Approval of Examining Boards in Dental Specialties of the ADA Council on Dental Education and Licensure.[49] The principal purposes of the Board, as defined in its Articles of Incorporation, are to protect and improve the public's health by the study and creation of standards for the practice of dental public health, grant and issue dental public health certificates to dentists who have successfully completed the prescribed training and experience requisite for the practice of dental public health, and ensure continuing competency of diplomates.[49]

Association of State and Territorial Dental Directors

The ASTDD is primarily made up of state dental directors and provides information and advocacy to the states and territories in the United States. The ASTDD supports programs and initiatives for community water fluoridation, school fluoride programs, school sealant programs, workforce development, special health care needs, and access to oral health services, which may include services to special groups, such as adults and seniors. The ASTDD helps develop state oral health surveillance systems, state oral health coalition, and oral health plans, and promotes best practices for state, territorial, and community oral health programs. The ASTDD is also an important resource for meeting the oral health objectives of Healthy People 2020.[50]

American Association of Community Dental Programs

The American Association of Community Dental Programs (AACDP) supports the efforts of those with an interest in serving the oral health needs at the community level. Members include local dental directors and staff of city-, county-, and community-based health programs. The AACDP has developed several publications to help local public health agencies incorporate oral health into public health services. These include "A Guide for Developing and Enhancing Community Oral Health Programs," "A Model Framework for Community Oral Health Programs Based Upon the Ten Essential Public Health Services," and "Seal America: The Prevention Invention."[51]

American Dental Education Association

The mission of the American Dental Education Association (ADEA) is to lead individuals and institutions of the dental education community to address contemporary issues influencing education, research, and the delivery of oral health care for the improvement of the health of the public.[52] ADEA has a section on community and preventive dentistry and behavioral sciences. ADEA also publishes the *Journal of Dental Education* and the *Bulletin of Dental Education*.

National Network on Oral Health Access

The National Network on Oral Health Access is a nationwide network of dental providers who care for patients in migrant, homeless, and community health centers. Members have displayed commitment to improving the health of the underserved through increased access to oral health services.[53]

DENTAL WORKFORCE ASSURANCE

Dental public health emphasizes the availability of a competent oral health workforce to serve the American population, with particular focus on ensuring access to dental care for traditionally underserved populations. The current dental workforce is predominated by dentists, dental hygienists, and dental assistants. However, dental therapists, community dental health workers, and other emerging provider models are becoming increasingly common.

Dentists

Since 2001, the US dentist workforce has increased by 20%, from 163,345 to 196,441 professionally active dentists.[7] This translates into a current dentist/population ratio of approximately 61 dentists per 100,000 Americans. However, wide geographic variation in dentist ratios exists: Arkansas has 41 dentists per 100,000 population, whereas the District of Columbia has 88.5 dentists per 100,000 population. It should be noted that these figures include dentists working in a variety of professional settings, including private practice, residencies, public health, research, and administration.

Ten new dental schools opened in the United States from 2008 to 2016,[54] for a total of 66 dental schools currently operating in the United States and 10 in Canada.[55] The number of dental graduates has increased consistently over the last decade, with 5811 new graduates in 2015.[55] After completion of a 4-year, university-based curriculum approved by CODA, dentists must pass national board examinations and fulfill a clinical examination as requirements for licensure. Licensure requirements vary by state. In several states, dentists may complete an accredited postgraduate dental education program in lieu of, or in addition to, a clinical licensure examination.[56] Dentists may choose to pursue additional education in an advanced education program for general practice or a dental specialty.

Most dentists (79.0%) are general practitioners. The three most common dental specialties include orthodontics (5.4% of practicing dentists), oral and maxillofacial surgery (3.9%), and pediatric dentistry (3.7%).[7] As the newest ADA-recognized dental specialty, oral and maxillofacial radiology has shown the greatest increased in workforce supply, from eight recognized specialists in 2001 to 116 in 2016. However, pediatric dentistry has also shown substantial growth, with that workforce increasing by 84% since 2001, with 7337 specialists in 2016.[7]

Recent changes in the US dentist workforce reflect national shifts in demographics and professional work patterns. As of 2016, women make up 30% of professionally active dentists in the United States, up from 16% in 2001, and dentists age 65 and older now make up 15% of the professionally active workforce.[7]

The US HRSA currently estimates that 8,323 dentists would be required to alleviate existing designated shortage areas.[57] However, this estimate does not necessarily indicate that there is an overall dentist shortage of this magnitude; workforce shortages can also be created by geographic maldistributions of dentists relative to the overall population.

Along with the resultant increases in dental graduates, retirements from the Baby Boomer generation will also begin to slow down over the coming decades. These changes are expected to contribute to an increased per capita supply of dentists in the United States through 2035, when dentist/population ratios are expected to be nearly 67 dentists per 100,000 population.[54] Increases in dentist supply are expected even if adjustments are made for expected reductions in the number of hours worked per dentist and reductions in patient visits per dentist.

Most private practitioners employ additional nondentist staff. In 2013, a total of 69% of dentists employed dental hygienists, 87% employed chairside assistants, and 20% employed expanded-function dental assistants.[58]

Dental Hygienists

As of 2014, there were 200,500 dental hygienists employed in the United States, with employment projected to grow 19% by 2024.[59] Hygienists are health care providers who must graduate from an accredited education program, complete a national written examination, and then obtain licensure by state or regional clinical examination. Dental hygiene education programs include certificate programs, associate's, bachelor's, and master's degree programs; most hygienists in the workforce have an associate's degree. There are currently 336 accredited education programs in the United States.[60]

Most hygienists work in private dental offices, where they typically provide prophylaxis, scaling and root planing, take radiographs, apply sealants, and provide topical fluoride treatment. However, they are also employed in a variety of other settings, including community-based public health settings, and work under various degrees of dentist supervision. Scope of practice and required level of dentist supervision are established by state law. Under direct supervision, a dentist is required to be physically present.[61] With general supervision, a dentist is required to have examined a patient or specifically authorized services to be provided without an examination.

Many states permit less supervision in certain public settings. In 2016, a total of 39 states permitted hygienists to provide preventive oral health services in community-based settings (eg, schools and nursing homes) without requiring direct or general supervision by a dentist.[60] Dental hygienists working under direct access requirement can assess patients and initiate treatment without the specific authorization of a dentist.[62] In 1995, five states permitted direct access; in 2016, a total of 39 states permitted some form of direct access for hygienists. Direct access models include collaborative agreements with a dentist, public health practice, and extended care permits. Typically, licensure for direct access has additional requirements, often including specified lengths of clinical experience, annual reporting, and carrying professional liability insurance.[63]

California's direct access model, the registered dental hygienist in alternative practice, allows hygienists to receive advanced licensure to provide unsupervised services in practice settings that are traditionally considered to be underserved: residential facilities, hospitals, dental health professional shortage areas, and residences of the homebound.[62] One study of alternative practice in California found that most patients treated by a registered dental hygienist in alternative practice were medically compromised or physically disabled.[64]

Dental Assistants

Dental assistants are also regulated at the state level, with allowable tasks and supervision requirements varying based on education and training.[65] Titles also vary by state, with certified dental assistants, registered dental assistants, and expanded function dental assistants; qualifications and scopes of practice vary considerably by state. In many states, dental hygienists may also apply for expanded duties as expanded function dental auxiliaries.

There are a variety of educational pathways for dental assistants, ranging from on-the-job training to formal training programs in community colleges, trade and technical schools, and dental schools. There are currently approximately 270 CODA-accredited dental assisting education programs in the United States. In 2014, these programs graduated a total of 5,756 dental assisting students.[65] Dental assistants may directly enter the workforce, although many states require additional credentialing or licensure to provide specific services.[65]

Recent national data indicate that there are approximately 300,000 jobs for dental assistants in the United State, with job growth projected to be 25% by 2022. Since 1990, the ratio of dental assistants per dentist has remained stable, with 1.7 assistants per dentist in 2012.[65]

Other Dental Providers

Other dental providers, often referred to as midlevel providers, include dental health aide therapists (DHATs) and dental therapists. Introduced by the Alaska Native Tribal Health Consortium in 2004 to provide care for Alaska Natives in tribal villages, DHATs were the first recognized dental therapists in the United States. The Alaska Dental Health Aide Initiative also introduced primary dental health aides, expanded function dental health aides, and dental health aid hygienists.[66] By 2013, there were 58 dental health aides in Alaska, including 25 DHATs.

The Alaska model is based on New Zealand's dental therapists, originally referred to as dental nurses. DHATs complete 2 years of education post–high school, complete a preceptorship, and are certified (rather than licensed) by Alaska's Community Health Aide/Practitioner Program. Curricula and standards are aligned with similar providers nationally and with dental therapy programs in other countries.[66]

The New Zealand model is now used in 54 countries.[67] A review of the global literature related to practice of dental therapists since inception of this model in 1921 found that most dental therapists are employed by government agencies to care for children, often in school-based programs.[67] Because their scope of practice is primarily limited to children, studies have found that dental therapists improve access to care for that population. Studies have also consistently found that dental therapists provide more economical care, with quality comparable with that of a dentist.[67] Dental therapists also have favorable patient and parent support in countries where they practice.

Minnesota legislation authorized the practice of dental therapy in 2009.[68] Originally, two programs were developed to educate dental therapists: a bachelor's program leading to licensure as a dental therapist, and a master of dental therapy program leading to licensure as an advanced dental therapist. Since their inception, both programs have been modified to provide the same curriculum. The bachelor's program is a 32-month full-time program, whereas the master's program is 16 months. Future Minnesota dental therapists will be dually licensed as dental therapists and dental hygienists.[68]

Dental therapists in Minnesota are primarily limited by legislation to practice in settings that serve low-income populations, the uninsured, or in shortage areas.[68] Dental therapists are required to work under a collaborative agreement with a licensed Minnesota dentist, with scope of practice and level of supervision currently varying for advanced dental therapists and dental therapists. By 2014, there were 32 licensed dental therapists in Minnesota.[69] A recent evaluation of Minnesota's dental therapists found that 84% of patients served by dental therapists were enrolled in public health insurance programs.[69] Patients reported reduced travel times, reduced wait times for dental care, and improved satisfaction with dental care.[70] Dental clinics that employ therapists report increased productivity, direct costs savings, improved patient satisfaction, and reduced broken appointment rates.[69]

Recently, Alaska's DHAT model has been expanded to American Indian tribes in Washington and Oregon, with several tribes in those states beginning pilot projects to hire dental therapists.[70] Currently, Maine and Vermont also recognize dental therapists as licensed providers; several states are considering legislation that would authorize dental therapy.[71]

SUMMARY

Dental public health is a unique specialty of dentistry where the focus is on the community rather than an individual, and on prevention rather than only treating existing disease. The target population is often vulnerable with poor access to the dental care delivery system, at higher risk of developing dental disease, and with limited resources at their disposal. This presents a complex and challenging problem that requires multipronged solutions borrowing constructs from multiple disciplines. As a result, dental public health professionals and their training are an amalgamation of diverse disciplines including but not limited to preventive dentistry, epidemiology, biostatistics, behavioral health, health economics, health policy, and health care administration. Although there are only 154 active board-certified public health dentists in the United States, the dental public health workforce extends beyond that to include other dentists, dental hygienists, and nondental professionals who are working to further the goal of this specialty. These professionals work at local, state, and national levels, and in private organizations to improve oral health and overall health of the population.

ACKNOWLEDGMENTS

The authors wish to acknowledge Myron Allukian and Olubunmi Adekugbe's previous article titled "The Practice and Infrastructure of Dental Public Health in the United States" published in a 2008 special issue of this journal (Allukian & Adekugbe, 2008). The current article offers an update and describes current dental public health practice and infrastructure in the United States.

REFERENCES

1. Tomar SL. An assessment of the dental public health infrastructure in the United States. J Public Health Dent 2006;66(1):5–16.

2. American Dental Association. Dental Public Health. Available at: http://www.ada.org/en/member-center/oral-health-topics/dental-public-health. Accessed June 14, 2017.

3. Winslow CE. The untilled fields of public health. Science 1920;23–33.

4. Institute of Medicine. The future of public health. Washington, DC: The National Academies Press; 1988.

5. Commission on Dental Accreditation. Accreditation standards for advanced specialty education programs in dental public health. Chicago: Commission on

Dental Accreditation; 2016. Available at: http://www.ada.org/~/media/CODA/Files/2017_dph.pdf?la=on. Accessed June 14, 2017.

6. WHO. Oral Health Factsheet. Available at: http://www.who.int/mediacentre/factsheets/fs318/en/. Accessed July 21, 2017.

7. FDI. Vision 2020 think tank: a new definition for oral health. Available at: http://www.fdiworlddental.org/sites/default/files/media/images/oral_health_definition-exec_summary-en.pdf. Accessed July 14, 2017.

8. ABDPH Newsletter 2017. Available at: https://aaphd.memberclicks.net/assets/ABDPH/Newsletters/ABDPHFall2017Newsletter.pdf. Accessed January, 2018.

9. Healthy Policy Institute. Supply of dentists in the U.S.: 2001-2016. Chicago: American Dental Association; 2017. Available at: http://www.ada.org/en/science-research/health-policy-institute/data-center/supply-and-profile-of-dentists. Accessed July 23, 2017.

10. Rozier RG. Proceedings: workshop to develop competency objectives in dental public health. J Public Health Dent 1990;50:330–44.

11. Dental public health competencies. J Public Health Dent 1998;58(S1):121–2.

12. Weintraub JA, Rozier GR. Updated competencies for the dental public health specialist: using the past and present to frame the future. J Public Health Dent 2016;76:S4–10.

13. Altman D, Mascarenhas AK. New competencies for the 21st century dental public health specialist. J Public Health Dent 2016;76:S18–28.

14. CDC. Ten Great Public Health Achievements in the 20th Century. Available at: https://www.cdc.gov/about/history/tengpha.htm. Accessed June 18, 2017.

15. Fisher-Owens SA, Gansky SA, Platt LJ, et al. Influences on children's oral health: a conceptual model. Pediatrics 2007;120:510–20.

16. Beauchamp DE. Public health as social justice. Inquiry 1976;13(1):3–14.

17. WHO. Constitution of the World Health Organization. 1946. Available at: http://www.who.int/governance/eb/who_constitution_en.pdf. Accessed June 18, 2017.

18. Health and Human Services. HHS FY 2017 budget in brief. Available at: https://www.hhs.gov/about/budget/fy2017/budget-in-brief/index.html?language=es. Accessed May 18, 2017.

19. Commissioned Corps of the US Public Health Service: Dental Professional Advisory Committee. US Public Health Service- Dental Category. Available at: https://dcp.psc.gov/osg/dentlst/. Accessed May 18, 2017.

20. Indian Health Service. Agency Overview. Available at: https://www.ihs.gov/aboutihs/overview/. Accessed May 18, 2017.

21. Batliner TS. Improving the oral health of American Indians and Alaska Natives. J Health Care Poor Underserved 2016;27(1A):1–10.

22. CDC Budget Request Overview. FY 2017 Presidents' Budget Request. Available at: https://www.cdc.gov/budget/documents/fy2017/cdc-overview-factsheet.pdf. Accessed May 18, 2017.

23. Oral Health Program Strategic Plan 2011-2014. Available at: https://www.cdc.gov/oralhealth/pdfs/oral_health_strategic_plan.pdf. Accessed May 18, 2017.

24. Healthy People 2020: Oral Health Objectives. Available at: https://www.healthypeople.gov/2020/topics-objectives/topic/oral-health/objectives. Accessed May 18, 2017.

25. National Institutes of Health. Budget. Available at: https://www.nih.gov/about-nih/what-we-do/budget. Accessed May 18, 2017.

26. National Institute of Dental and Craniofacial Research. About US. Available at: https://www.nidcr.nih.gov/AboutUs/FastFacts.htm. Accessed May 18, 2017.

27. Health Resources and Service Administration. Available at: https://www.hrsa.gov/about/index.html. Accessed June 12, 2017.

28. Health Resources and Service Administration. Oral Health. Available at: https://www.hrsa.gov/oralhealth/. Accessed June 10, 2017.

29. Ryan White & Global HIV/AIDS Programs. Health Resources and Administration. Available at: https://hab.hrsa.gov/about-ryan-white-hivaids-program/part-f-dental-programs. Accessed June 12, 2017.

30. Ryan White & Global HIV/AIDS Programs. Oral Health and HIV. Available at: https://www.hrsa.gov/publichealth/clinical/oralhealth/hivfactsheet.pdf. Accessed June 12, 2017.

31. HRSA. National Health Service Corps. Available at: https://www.nhsc.hrsa.gov/. Accessed May 18, 2017.

32. National Health Service Corps. An overview of the dental health care provider shortage. Available at: https://nhsc.hrsa.gov/downloads/nhscdentalhealth.pdf. Accessed May 18, 2017.

33. Centers for Medicare and Medicaid Services. Available at: https://www.cms.gov/about-cms/about-cms.html. Accessed May 28, 2017.

34. Dental Care. Medicaid.gov. Available at: https://www.medicaid.gov/medicaid/benefits/dental/index.html. Accessed May 28, 2017.

35. CMS. Update on CMS Oral Health Initiative and Other Oral Health Related Item. Available at: https://www.medicaid.gov/federal-policy-guidance/downloads/cib-07-10-2014.pdf. Accessed May 28, 2017.

36. CMS. Medicare Program- General Information. Available at: https://www.cms.gov/Medicare/Medicare-General-Information/MedicareGenInfo/index.html. Accessed May 26, 2017.

37. Agency for Healthcare Research and Quality. Available at: https://www.ahrq.gov/cpi/about/profile/index.html. Accessed May 18, 2017.

38. AHRQ. Dental Plan. Available at: https://www.ahrq.gov/cahps/surveys-guidance/dental/index.html. Accessed May 18, 2017.

39. AHRQ Oral Health Resources. Available at: https://www.ahrq.gov/research/findings/final-reports/oral-health/index.html. Accessed May 18, 2017.

40. Tomar SL. Assessment of the Dental Public Health Infrastructure in the United States. 2004. Available at: https://www.nidcr.nih.gov/DataStatistics/Documents/US_Dental_Public_Health_Infrastructure_8_2004.pdf. Accessed June 10, 2017.

41. Association of State and Territorial Dental Directors. 2016 synopses of State Dental Public Health Programs: Data for FY 2014-2015. Available at: http://www.astdd.org/docs/synopses-report-summary-2016.pdf. Accessed June 12, 2017.

42. Operational definition of a functional local health department (NACCHO). 2005. Available at: http://www.naccho.org/uploads/downloadable-resources/OperationalDefinitionBrochure-2.pdf. Accessed June 17, 2017.

43. 2016 National Profile of Local Health Departments (NACCHO). Available at: http://nacchoprofilestudy.org/wp-content/uploads/2017/04/ProfileReport_Final3b.pdf. Accessed June 28, 2017.

44. Edelstein B. The dental safety net, its workforce, and policy recommendations for its enhancement. J Public Health Dent 2010;70:s1.

45. Vujicic M, Buchmueller T, Klein R. Dental care presents the highest level of financial barriers, compared to other types of health care services. Health Aff 2016; 35(12):2176–82.

46. America's Health Centers. Fact Sheet March 2016 by National Association of Community Health Centers. Available at: http://www.nachc.org/wp-content/

uploads/2015/06/Americas-Health-Centers-March-2016.pdf. Accessed June 19, 2017.

47. Oral Health: American Public Health Association. Available at: https://www.apha.org/apha-communities/member-sections/oral-health. Accessed June 22, 2017.

48. About the AAPHD. Available at: http://www.aaphd.org/. Accessed June 22, 2017.

49. American Board of Dental Public Health. Available at: http://www.aaphd.org/abdph. Accessed June 22, 2017.

50. Association of State and Territorial Dental Directors. Available at: http://www.astdd.org/. Accessed June 22, 2017.

51. American Association for Community Dental Programs. Available at: https://www.aacdp.com/. Accessed June 22, 2017.

52. American Dental Education Association. Available at: http://www.adea.org/. Accessed June 22, 2017.

53. National Network for Oral Health Access. Available at: http://www.nnoha.org/. Accessed June 22, 2017.

54. Munson B, Vujicic M. Number of practicing dentists per capita in the United States will grow steadily. Chicago: ADA Health Policy Institute; 2016. Available at: http://www.ada.org/~/media/ADA/Science%20and%20Research/HPI/Files/HPIBrief_0616_1.pdf?la=en. Accessed July 23, 2017.

55. American Dental Education Association. 2016. ADEA Snapshot of Dental Education, 2016-2017. Washington, DC. Available at: http://www.adea.org/snapshot/. Accessed July 23, 2017.

56. American Dental Association. State Licensure for US Dentists. Chicago (IL). Available at: http://www.ada.org/en/education-careers/licensure/state-dental-licensure-for-us-dentists. Accessed July 23, 2017.

57. HRSA Data Warehouse. 2017. Designated Health Professional Shortage Areas Statistics. Available at: https://datawarehouse.hrsa.gov/topics/shortageAreas.aspx. Accessed July 23, 2017.

58. Health Policy Institute. 2013 Employment of dental practice personnel. Chicago: American Dental Association; 2015. Table 1. Available at: http://www.ada.org/en/science-research/health-policy-institute/data-center/dental-practice. Accessed July 23, 2017.

59. Bureau of Labor Statistics, U.S. Department of Labor. Occupational Outlook Handbook, 2016-17 edition, Dental Hygienists. Available at: https://www.bls.gov/ooh/healthcare/dental-hygienists.htm. Accessed July 23, 2017.

60. American Dental Hygienists' Association. Facts about the dental hygiene workforce in the United States. 2016. Available at: https://www.adha.org/resources-docs/75118_Facts_About_the_Dental_Hygiene_Workforce.pdf. Accessed July 23, 2017.

61. National Governors Association. The role of dental hygienists in providing access to oral health care. Washington, DC. 2014. Available at: https://www.nga.org/files/live/sites/NGA/files/pdf/2014/1401DentalHealthCare.pdf. Accessed July 23, 2017.

62. American Dental Hygienists' Association. ADHA Policy Manual [4S-09]. Chicago (IL). 2016. Available at: http://www.adha.org/resources-docs/7614_Policy_Manual.pdf. Accessed July 23, 2017.

63. American Dental Hygienists' Association. Direct access to care from dental hygienists. Chicago (IL). 2017. Available at: http://www.adha.org/resources-docs/7513_Direct_Access_to_Care_from_DH.pdf. Accessed July 23, 2017.

64. Mertz E, Glassman P. Alternative practice dental hygiene in California: past, present, and future. J Calif Dent Assoc 2011;39(1):37–46.

65. Baker B, Langelier M, Moore J, et al. The dental assistant workforce in the United States, 2015. Rensselaer (NY): Center for Health Workforce Studies, School of Public Health, SUNY Albany; 2015.
66. Shoffstall-Cone S, WIlliard M. Alaska dental health aide program. Int J Circumpolar Health 2013;72:21198.
67. Nash DA, Friedman JW, Mathu-Muju KR, et al. A review of the global literature on dental therapists. Community Dent Oral Epidemiol 2013;42(1):1–10.
68. Self K, Brickle C. Dental therapy education in Minnesota. Am J Public Health 2017;107(S1):S77–80.
69. Minnesota Department of Health. Minnesota Board of Dentistry. Early impacts of dental therapists in Minnesota. Report to the Minnesota Legislature 2014. 2014. Available at: http://www.health.state.mn.us/divs/orhpc/workforce/dt/dtlegisrpt. pdf. Accessed July 23, 2017.
70. Grant J, Myszka N. Oregon dental pilot to expand tribes' access to care. Midlevel providers to join clinic teams. The Pew Charitable Trusts; 2016. Available at: http://www.pewtrusts.org/en/research-and-analysis/analysis/2016/02/11/oregon-dental-pilot-to-expand-tribes-access-to-care. Accessed July 23, 17.
71. Koppelman J. States expand the use of dental therapy. Philadelphia: The Pew Charitable Trusts; 2016. Available at: http://www.pewtrusts.org/en/research-and-analysis/analysis/2016/09/28/states-expand-the-use-of-dental-therapy. Accessed July 23, 2017.

Oral Health Disparities Across the Life Span

Michelle M. Henshaw, DDS, MPH[a,b,c,*], Raul I. Garcia, DMD, MMedSc[b,c], Jane A. Weintraub, DDS, MPH[d]

KEYWORDS

- Oral health • Health status disparities • Social determinants of health
- Vulnerable populations • Epidemiology

KEY POINTS

- Oral health disparities in the United States are profound and individuals from low-income and minority populations tend to bear the greatest burden of oral diseases.
- It is vital that members of the dental profession understand the distribution of oral health and disease across different populations and the life span. There are few absolute patterns in the epidemiology of oral health disparities, with the exception of poverty. Poor individuals almost universally experience a greater burden of oral diseases and conditions than those with more resources. Individuals from racial and ethnic minority groups, in particular Native Americans, Alaskan Natives, Blacks, and Hispanics also generally experience higher levels of dental caries, periodontal disease, tooth loss, and orofacial pain as well as oral cancer incidence and survival rates than non-Hispanic Whites.
- Although the country has made strides to reduce some of the disparities originally described in *Oral Health in America: A Report of the Surgeon General*, released in 2000, much work remains.
- Unfortunately, many low-income, low-educated, and disadvantaged populations with the highest levels of untreated dental disease are the very people who lack access to high-quality care for the multitude of reasons outlined in this article. Importantly, many of these factors are under practitioners' control, so there is hope that by working collaboratively as individual practitioners and through dental societies and other dental and health professional organizations it is possible to bring an end to oral health disparities can be brought about in the United States.

Continued

Disclosures: The authors have identified no professional or financial affiliations for themselves or their spouse/partner.
[a] Office of Global and Population Health, Boston University Henry M. Goldman School of Dental Medicine, 560 Harrison Avenue, 3rd Floor, Boston, MA 02118, USA; [b] Department of Health Policy & Health Services Research, Boston University Henry M. Goldman School of Dental Medicine, 560 Harrison Avenue, 3rd Floor, Boston, MA 02118, USA; [c] Center for Research to Evaluate and Eliminate Dental Disparities (CREEDD), Boston University Henry M. Goldman School of Dental Medicine, 560 Harrison Avenue, Boston, MA 02118, USA; [d] UNC School of Dentistry, The University of North Carolina at Chapel Hill, Koury Oral Health Sciences Building, Room 4508, Chapel Hill, North Carolina 27599-7450
* Corresponding author. Office of Global and Population Health, Boston University Henry M. Goldman School of Dental Medicine, 560 Harrison Avenue, 3rd Floor, Boston, MA 02118.
E-mail address: mhenshaw@bu.edu

Dent Clin N Am 62 (2018) 177–193
https://doi.org/10.1016/j.cden.2017.12.001
0011-8532/18/© 2017 Elsevier Inc. All rights reserved.

dental.theclinics.com

Continued

- Oral health professionals must also actively advocate for incorporation of oral health into now and existing health policy and form stronger alliances with the other health professions and health professional organizations to ensure optimal oral health for all populations.

INTRODUCTION

Good oral health is essential to overall health and well-being throughout life. Despite improvements in the oral health status of the United States population as a whole, a disproportionately higher burden of oral diseases and disorders are still borne by certain segments of the population. These differences in health status, health outcomes, or health care use between distinct socially disadvantaged and advantaged groups are known as health disparities. The definition of health disparity used by *Healthy People 2020* is "... a particular type of health difference that is closely linked with social, economic, social, and/or environmental disadvantage. Health disparities adversely affect groups of people who have systematically experienced greater obstacles to health based on their racial or ethnic group; religion; socioeconomic status; gender; age; mental health; cognitive, sensory, or physical disability; sexual orientation or gender identity; geographic location; or other characteristics historically linked to discrimination or exclusion."[1]

Outside the United States, the term, *health inequalities*, is more commonly used than health disparities. Whitehead[2] defined health inequalities as health differences that are avoidable, unnecessary, and unjust. Not all health differences are avoidable, such as prostate cancer in men versus in women, or unjust, such as a difference in the proportion of basketball and nonbasketball players who have had sprained ankles. The unjust component pertains to the human rights principle of health equity, that people should not be denied health or health care because they belong to a particular group.[3] Braveman[4] points out that equal treatment may still be unjust if some disadvantaged groups need and do not receive more resources or services than others to be healthy. For example, a short child might need a stepstool to reach the sink to brush her teeth, a resource not needed by someone taller, but both should have toothbrushing opportunity (**Fig. 1**).

At the request of Congress, the Institute of Medicine (now the Health and Medicine Division of the National Academies of Sciences, Engineering, and Medicine) explored why racial and ethnic disparities in health care exist, even when other factors, such as income, access to care, and insurance coverage, are comparable and found that "bias, discrimination, and stereotyping at the provider, patient, institutional, and health system levels..."[5] contribute to disparities. These findings were published in the report, *Unequal Treatment: Confronting Racial and Ethnic Disparities in Health Care*, in 2002.[5] Almost a decade later, the US Department of Health and Human Services 2011 report, *HHS Action Plan to Reduce Racial and Ethnic Health Disparities*,[6] described health disparities between ethnic minority populations and Whites. These disparities include differences in access to care, preventive care, preventable hospitalizations, poorer overall health, and more severe forms of serious illness and are influenced by a diverse set of factors. For example, many American adults have limited English proficiency that exacerbates their inability to navigate the health care system and adhere to treatment recommendations.[7] Recent research has also explored some of the underlying biologic pathways of social determinants of health. For example,

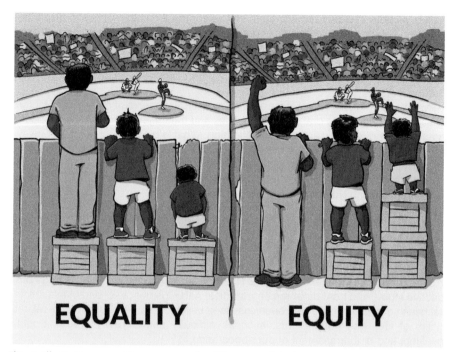

EQUALITY   **EQUITY**

Fig. 1. Illustrating equality versus equity. (*Courtesy of* Artist, Angus Maguire, Interaction Institute for Social Change. Available at: interactioninstitute.org and madewithangus. com; with permission.)

chronic stress can disrupt immune systems, trigger inflammatory mediators, shorten telomeres, or, in childhood, alter neural development.[4]

As described in this article, disparities also apply to oral health and these are among the most profound health disparities in the United States.[8] It is vital that members of the dental profession understand the distribution of oral health and disease across different populations and the life span and participate in developing innovative and sustainable approaches to eliminate oral health disparities. This is challenging because there are few absolute patterns in the epidemiology of oral health disparities, with the exception of poverty. Poor individuals almost universally experience a greater burden of oral diseases and conditions than those with more resources. Individuals from racial and ethnic minority groups, in particular Native Americans, Alaskan Natives, Blacks, and Hispanics, also generally experience higher levels of dental caries, periodontal disease, tooth loss, and orofacial pain as well as oral cancer incidence and survival rates than non-Hispanic Whites.

To understand the root causes of oral health disparities it is necessary to recognize the role of the social determinants of health: factors such as where people live, their environment, income, education and health literacy level, and social support. These factors in turn influence biological and genetic expression and behavioral factors related to oral disease and are subsequently impacted by differential access to health care for prevention and treatment. Access to dental care is influenced by public policies, insurance coverage, availability of providers who accept that insurance and speak the same language, out-of-pocket affordability, transportation, ability to take time off from work, cultural norms, and perceived need. These factors exist at the individual, family, and community levels and their complex interplay contributes to the challenges both in understanding their relative contributions to oral health disparities and in developing effective models to prevent oral diseases. It is well recognized, however, that by addressing the underlying, higher-order, upstream factors contributing to poor oral health, such as poverty and safe affordable housing, that reductions in oral health disparities are more likely than if the focus continues to be on treating disease after it occurs.[9]

Given this complexity, it is not surprising the interrelationship of many of the factors believed to contribute to oral health disparities and their relative impact are still poorly understood and require additional investigation. What is clearly documented, however, is the oral health status as measured by calibrated examiners who conducted examinations in mobile centers, using structured clinical examination protocols in national representative samples of the US population, conducted as part of the ongoing National Health and Nutrition Examination Survey (NHANES). In the next few sections, NHANES[10] data are used to provide information about the unequal distribution of the major oral diseases and conditions—dental caries, periodontal disease, and tooth loss in the United States. Information about oral cancer comes primarily from Surveillance, Epidemiology, and End Results (SEER) Program of the National Cancer Institute.[11] Some of the data on orofacial pain and temporomandibular disorder (TMD) are based on self-reports collected in the National Health Interview Survey (NHIS),[12] a large prospective study, and from other regional studies. Although not described in this article, oral health disparities have also been assessed using measures of oral health–related quality of life, with components, such as difficulty chewing, dry mouth, trouble speaking, and embarrassment about appearance.[13]

DENTAL CARIES

Although there have been dramatic reductions in the prevalence of dental caries in the United States over the past several decades, caries remains a significant public health problem, and substantial disparities remain in both racial and ethnic minority groups and financially disadvantaged groups. These disparities persist throughout the life span, despite simple preventive strategies, such as fluoride in different formats and dental sealants, which are effective in preventing this disease, especially if caries risk factors, such as poor oral hygiene, sugary diet, and reduced salivary flow, often a result of medications, are reduced.

Children

Caries is the most common chronic childhood condition in the United States. According to the most recent NHANES data available (2011–2014), the overall prevalence of caries experience (treated plus untreated caries) in children (2–19 years old) has not significantly changed since the last wave of data collection that took place in 1999 to 2004. These data were collected using mirrors and explorers for caries detection. Visual evidence alone of demineralization was not considered to be caries and no radiographs were exposed; thus, disease prevalence and severity may be underestimated.[10] The assessment criteria for caries detection has been stable over time, however, and although the data may be conservative estimates of caries, the trends reported are accurate.

For children aged 2 years to 5 years, caries experience in the primary dentition declined from 27.7% to 23.8% and for those aged 6 years to 8 years, the overall prevalence increased from 51.5% to 52.8%; however, neither of these changes was statistically significant (**Table 1**). In children aged 2 years to 5 years from the lowest income groups, however, caries experience did significantly decline from 41.5% to

Table 1
Trends for dental caries in the primary and permanent dentition for children aged 2 years to 19 years

Category	Age Group (y)	1999–2004		2011–2014	
		%	SE	%	SE
Caries experience	2–5 y[a]	27.7	1.3	23.8	1.5
	6–8 y[a]	51.5	2.4	52.8	2.3
	2–8 y[a]	37.9	1.5	36.2	1.7
	6–8 y[b]	10.2	1.0	10.3	1.2
	9–11 y[b]	31.5	1.5	25.9	1.7[c]
	6–11 y[b]	20.9	0.9	18.2	1.1
	12–15 y[b]	50.7	1.2	48.2	2.0
	16–19 y[b]	67.5	1.4	66.6	1.7
	12–19 y[b]	59.4	1.0	57.7	1.4
Untreated caries	2–5 y[a]	20.4	1.2	11.0	1.0[c]
	6–8 y[a]	27.8	2.0	17.4	1.7[c]
	2–8 y[a]	23.5	1.4	13.7	1.1[c]
	6–8 y[b]	4.0	0.7	3.4	0.6
	9–11 y[b]	11.1	1.3	8.4	1.0
	6–11 y[b]	7.6	0.8	5.9	0.6
	12–15 y[b]	16.9	1.0	14.5	1.2
	16–19 y[b]	22.4	1.4	22.5	1.9
	12–19 y[b]	19.7	1.1	18.6	1.3

Source: National Health and Nutrition Examination Survey[10]; estimates for the 1999 through 2004 period and the 2011 through 2014 period were adjusted by single years of age from the 2010 US population.
[a] Primary teeth only.
[b] Permanent teeth only.
[c] $P<.05$.
Data from Dye BA, Mitnik GL, Iafolla TJ, et al. Trends in dental caries in children and adolescents according to poverty status in the United States from 1999 through 2004 and from 2011 through 2014. J Am Dent Assoc 2017;128(8):550–65.

34.7%. Although disparities in race and ethnicity persisted in 2011 to 2014, the prevalence of caries experience also showed nonsignificant declines in the 2-year to 5-year age group in all racial and ethnic groups (**Table 2**). Within these same racial and ethnic groups, if only those children 2 years to 5 years of age living below the federal poverty level are considered, the same pattern was evident, and although the caries experience in each group declined, non-Hispanic Whites had the greatest and only statistically significant decline from 40.6% to 26.1% (see **Table 2**). Therefore, despite improvements seen across all groups, disparities persisted, and in the case of the US, the youngest, poorest, most vulnerable children worsened because the relative gaps actually increased.[14]

Dental caries can have a negative impact on children's quality of life, lead to serious illness, and necessitate costly therapeutic interventions, such as treatment in the operating room under general anesthesia. The bacteria affecting primary teeth can affect the subsequent permanent dentition, and premature loss of primary teeth can affect the proper development and positioning of permanent teeth. The national public health agenda, as stated in Healthy People 2020, includes the goal to reduce the prevalence of children 3 years to 5 years old with dental caries experience in their primary teeth to 30% or less.[15] Based on the 2011 to 2014 data for 2 year olds to 5 year olds, it seems that this Healthy People 2020 objective may have already been achieved. When 2 year olds who are more likely to be caries-free are excluded, however, the

Table 2
Trends for dental caries in the primary and permanent dentition for US children aged 2 years to 19 years by poverty status and race/ethnicity

Category	Age Group	Poverty Status	Total 1999–2004 %	SE	Total 2011–2014 %	SE	Hispanic 1999–2004 %	SE	Hispanic 2011–2014 %	SE	Non-Hispanic Black 1999–2004 %	SE	Non-Hispanic Black 2011–2014 %	SE	Non-Hispanic White 1999–2004 %	SE	Non-Hispanic White 2011–2014 %	SE
Caries experience	2–5 y[a]	<100% FPG	41.5	2.2	34.7	1.9c	44.8	3.3	38.8	2.9	37.7	3.1	36.8	3.3	40.6	4.7	26.1	3.8
		100%–199% FPG	30.2	3.2	24.1	2.9	38.4	3.4	33.5	2.9	27.2	4.2	23.7	3.9	27.6	4.8	18.4	5.0
		≥200% FPG	17.7	1.5	16.5	2.3	20.7	2.8	14.5	3.0	22.9	2.9	16.0	4.1	15.9	1.8	16.6	3.
		Total	27.7	1.3	23.8	1.5	36.2	2.1	30.5	2.1	31.4	2.2	29.5	2.6	23.6	1.8	18.5	2.
	6–11 y[b]	<100% FPG	28.1	2.3	23.7	2.2	36.5	3.1	26.1	2.4d	20.3	2.2	28.0	2.9d	29.7	4.9	18.1	5.6
		100%–199% FPG	24.0	2.1	20.4	2.3	28.6	3.1	22.5	3.8	20.5	2.4	21.3	2.9	21.8	3.7	17.2	3.3
		≥200% FPG	16.2	1.3	13.4	1.6	19.9	2.6	18.4	3.8	14.1	2.8	13.2	2.9	15.6	1.6	12.6	2.2
		Total	20.9	0.9	18.2	1.1	28.7	1.7	22.7	2.4d	18.9	1.5	22.3	1.9	18.6	1.4	15.2	1.5
	12–19 y[b]	<100% FPG	65.8	1.4	65.6	2.3	70.3	2.6	68.5	3.0	57.0	2.5	65.5	3.0	66.5	2.7	66.1	3.3
		100%–199% FPG	64.7	1.5	66.0	2.7	62.4	2.5	65.8	4.5	53.9	2.7	58.6	3.5	69.1	2.7	69.5	4.3
		≥200% FPG	54.3	1.5	49.5	2.3	61.0	2.8	52.8	3.8	52.0	2.5	48.9	3.5	53.3	1.8	49.1	2.7
		Total	59.4	1.0	57.7	1.4	64.8	1.8	64.5	2.4	54.7	1.7	57.8	1.9	58.1	1.6	55.6	2.0
Untreated caries	2–5 y[a]	<100% FPG	31.1	1.9	17.6	2.1	34.0	3.0	20.1	3.0	29.1	3.1	21.2	3.0	29.5	4.1	11.2	3.2
		100%–199% FPG	22.9	3.0	11.0	1.6	28.9	3.7	17.9	3.6	20.5	4.0	11.8	2.7	20.4	4.2	6.9	2.3d
		≥200% FPG	12.8	1.2	6.2	1.0	13.0	2.0	8.3	1.8	18.6	3.1	DSU	DSU	11.4	1.3	5.4	1.3
		Total	20.4	1.2	11.0	1.0c	26.6	1.8	16.9	1.7	24.2	2.1	15.7	2.2	16.8	1.6	6.5	1.0
	6–11 y[b]	<100% FPG	11.7	1.7	8.4	0.9	11.4	1.3	10.0	1.7	10.5	1.7	9.2	1.9	12.0	4.0	6.3	1.9
		100%–199% FPG	11.8	1.9	6.3	1.6	14.4	3.2	7.9	2.1	9.7	1.9	5.3	1.3	9.7	2.7	DSU	DSU
		≥200% FPG	3.6	0.7	4.3	0.8	8.0	1.7	7.2	2.8	4.6	1.4	4.5	1.6	2.9	0.8	3.9	1.0
		Total	7.6	0.8	5.9	0.6	11.8	1.4	8.5	1.2	8.7	1.0	6.9	1.1	5.6	1.2	4.7	0.8
	12–19 y[b]	<100% FPG	27.2	2.0	25.9	2.0	31.3	2.3	20.7	3.1	31.2	1.7	28.0	3.3	24.0	3.8	31.7	5.4
		100%–199% FPG	27.1	1.8	22.6	2.2	29.2	2.8	24.3	3.6	26.4	2.7	22.5	3.3	26.3	2.7	23.0	3.0
		≥200% FPG	13.0	1.4	12.3	1.8	18.5	2.7	13.6	2.9	19.3	1.7	18.7	4.5	11.1	1.6	11.8	2.3
		Total	19.7	1.1	18.6	1.3	27.2	1.6	20.1	2.4	26.0	1.4	23.0	2.5	16.1	1.5	17.8	2.0

Source: National Health and Nutrition Examination Survey[1a]; estimates for the 1999 through 2004 period and the 2011 through 2014 period were adjusted by single years of age from the 2010 US population.

Abbreviations: DSU, data statistically unreliable (relative standard error ≥40%); FPG, federal poverty guidelines.

[a] Primary teeth.

[b] Permanent teeth.

[c] $P<.05$.

[d] Estimate should be interpreted with caution (relative standard error ≥30% but <40%).

Data from Dye BA, Mitnik GL, Iafolla TJ, et al. Trends in dental caries in children and adolescents according to poverty status in the United States from 1999 through 2004 and from 20 through 2014. J Am Dent Assoc 2017;128(8):550–65.

percentage of children with caries in the 3-year to 5-year age group will most likely be higher. In 2011 to 14, 35% of all 2 year olds to 5 year olds living below the federal poverty level had caries experience. Thus, even if the target is reached in the general population, it is unlikely that all population groups will achieve this important milestone.

When examining permanent dentition, the caries experience was 10% in children aged 6 years to 8 years, but the percentage more than doubled (26%) for children aged 9 years to 11 years and more than doubled again for 12 year olds to 19 year olds (58%)[14] (see **Table 1**). Because caries experience is a cumulative measure of disease in permanent teeth, this increase in prevalence of dental caries with age is expected, but the magnitude of the increase remains a concern. Following the same patterns seen in primary teeth, the prevalence of caries experience in permanent teeth was significantly higher among Hispanic children aged 6 years to 11 years (23%) and non-Hispanic Black children (22%) compared with non-Hispanic White children (15%) (see **Table 2**).The racial and ethnic disparities, however, seen in younger children were not as seen during adolescence (12–19 years of age). Caries experience was 56%, 58% and 65% in non-Hispanic White, non-Hispanic Black and Hispanic children, respectively, but these percentages were not significantly different[14] (see **Table 2**).

Another measure of dental caries is untreated tooth decay. Similar to caries experience, at a population level there has been a decrease in the prevalence of untreated caries in primary teeth over time (see **Table 1**). In data from 1999 to 2004, 24% of children aged 2 years to 8 years had untreated caries in their primary teeth, compared with 14% measured a decade later.[14] When comparing older NHANES oral health data (1974–1994 to 1999–2004), oral health disparities in untreated caries in children significantly increased. In the most recent data, these racial and ethnic disparities persisted; untreated tooth decay in primary teeth was significantly higher for both non-Hispanic Black (20%) and Hispanic (20%) children compared with non-Hispanic White children aged 2 years to 8 years (9%). In older children, 20% of adolescents aged 12 years to 19 years had untreated caries. Unlike in younger children, there were no significant differences in the prevalence of untreated caries in adolescents by race and ethnicity, although the prevalence was higher among non-Hispanic Black adolescents (23%) compared with Hispanic (20%) or non-Hispanic White (18%) adolescents.[14]

As discussed previously, both caries experience and untreated caries are impacted by poverty status (based on federal poverty guidelines that used family income and family size), and in 2001 to 2004, in children aged 2 years to 12 years there was approximately a 3-fold increase in the percent of untreated decay from children from the lowest income category (33.4%) to those in the highest income (12.5%)[16] (see **Table 2**). In a study to assess trends in the impact of income of untreated dental decay in children, NHANES data were analyzed, which were collected at 3 separate time points spanning 3 decades (1974–2004). Disparities in untreated caries by income were present at each of the 3 time points and, more importantly, despite population-wide declines in untreated caries during that time frame, absolute inequality slightly increased, whereas the relative disparities significantly increased.[16] In the most recent NHANES data, disparity by income persists but has decreased to approximately a 2-fold increase in untreated caries in children from the highest to lowest income category in children in all 3 age groups (primary teeth in 2–8 year olds and permanent teeth in 6–11 year olds and 12–19 year olds).[14]

Adults

Of all dentate adults age 20 years to 64 years, 91% had experienced dental caries and more than 1 in 4 (27%) had untreated decay, which translates to 53 million adults with unmet dental needs.[17] Although caries prevalence increased slightly with age, there was little variation in prevalence of untreated decay by age. Racial disparities were present, but in contrast to children, non-Hispanic White adults, individuals with higher incomes and those with more education had more overall caries experience. Untreated decay followed the same patterns seen in children with untreated tooth decay, more prevalent among Hispanic and non-Hispanic Black adults compared with non-Hispanic White and Asian adults. The 2011 to 2012 NHANE data also reveal disparities by education, with 41.5% of adults in this age range with less than high school education having untreated caries compared with 16.7% among those with more than high school education.[18] One of the *Healthy People 2020* objectives is to reduce the proportion of 35-year-old to 44-year-old adults with any untreated decay to 25% and it seems that the nation will likely reach that goal for the overall population, but again certain population groups, especially those with low education levels, will likely not meet the target.[19]

Elders

Although some oral health disparities related to caries also existed for older adults, according to the 2011 to 2012 NHANES data, these disparities are less marked than what are seen in the other age groups, possibly because those with worse oral health over time have become edentulous. Dental caries experience was nearly ubiquitous in those 65 and older (96%) who were dentate and the prevalence was consistent across all elders when comparing those 65 years to 74 years with those over 75 years of age. Racial and ethnic disparities did exist, however, mirroring what was seen in the younger adult population, with coronal caries prevalence higher among older non-Hispanic White adults compared with older non-Hispanic Black and Hispanic adults. In individuals 65 years old and older, Hispanics (39%) had the highest prevalence of untreated coronal tooth decay, followed by non-Hispanic Blacks (33%) and non-Hispanic Whites (16%).[19] Similar trends were seen in untreated root caries in individuals 75 and older. Hispanics (56.6%) had the highest prevalence of untreated root tooth decay, followed by non-Hispanic Blacks (52.2%) and 36.4% in non-Hispanic Whites. Previous data have shown that for those ages 65 years and older, rates of untreated coronal caries were highest among the poor (41.3%) and near poor (22.5%) versus nonpoor (15.3%), demonstrating an approximately 3-fold difference between the highest and lowest groups.[20]

TOOTH LOSS

When assessing trends in complete and partial tooth loss in adults over 50 years old using NHANES data from 1988 to 1994 and 2001 to 2004, an overall decrease in both the number of teeth lost (8.19–6.50) and rates of total edentulism (24.6% to 17.4%) was found. There were significant disparities across age, race/ethnicity, years of education, and levels of income. Increasing age, being Black, having fewer years of education, and lower income were factors associated with higher risk of being edentulous and, in dentate individuals, of having more missing teeth. In both complete and partial tooth loss, disparities were seen over time; however, the trends differed by condition. Disparities in income and age decreased during the 2 time points when assessing edentulism. In contrast, income and age disparities increased when comparing changes in partial tooth loss during the 2 time periods, but racial disparities decreased.[21]

Complete tooth loss is now largely a condition of those 65 and older. Only half of all adults aged 20 years to 64 years, however, retained all of their dentition (with the exception of third molars)[22] and from 2004 to 2009 the average number of retained teeth in this age group was 25.[23] When limiting the data to older adults, the prevalence of edentulism rises to 19% of adults who are ages 65 years and over and increases with age, becoming twice as prevalent among adults aged 75 years and over (26%) compared with those aged 65 years to 74 years (13%). There is virtually no difference when comparing genders; however, there are disparities by race and ethnicity. Non-Hispanic Black adults over 65 years of age were more likely to be edentulous (29%) compared with older non-Hispanic Whites (17%) or Hispanic adults (15%).[22] Disparities were also seen by level of education; of those ages 65 years to 74 years with less than high school education, 29% were edentulous, approximately 2 times worse than those with more than a high school education (7%).[24] Complete tooth loss is an area where it seems that both the general population and all of the racial and ethnic groups will achieve the *Healthy People 2020* target of having no more than 21.6% of population be edentulous.[24]

PERIODONTAL DISEASE

Like dental caries, periodontal disease is a substantial public health problem and is not distributed evenly among the US adult population. Using NHANES data from 2009 through 2012, Eke and colleagues[25,26] estimated that approximately half (47%) of the US population over 30 years of age, or approximately 65 million adults, were afflicted with periodontal disease, as defined by the Centers for Disease Control/American Association of Periodontology case definitions for surveillance of periodontitis.[25,26] Among the afflicted population, the vast majority (83%) had nonsevere periodontal disease, which is either mild or moderate cases of periodontitis, whereas 17% had severe disease.[27]

Like caries, the likelihood of periodontal disease increased with age and also differed based on race and ethnicity. There were also gender disparities. After adjusting for age, men had a higher prevalence of periodontal disease when compared with women (57% vs 39%). Compared with non-Hispanic Whites, periodontal disease was more likely in Hispanics (adjusted prevalence rate [aPR] = 1.38; 95% CI, 1.26–1.52) and non-Hispanic Blacks (aPR = 1.35; 95% CI, 1.22–1.50), whereas severe periodontal disease was most likely in non-Hispanic Blacks (aPR = 1.82; 95% CI, 1.44–2.31). Individuals with less than a high school education were more likely to have both severe periodontal disease (aPR = 1.63; 95% CI, 1.26–2.12) and nonsevere periodontal disease (aPR = 1.29; 95% CI, 1.15–1.45) compared with those with greater than a high school education. Income status showed the same trend, an increase in likelihood of disease as poverty level increased. The highest probability for severe periodontal disease was seen in adults with the middle-income category 100% to 199% of federal poverty level (FPL) (aPR = 1.82; 95% CI, 1.22–2.71); in contrast, the highest probability for nonsevere periodontal disease was seen in the lowest income category (less than 100 FPL) (aPR = 1.44; 95% CI, 1.26–1.56). Current smoking status also significantly increased risk for periodontal disease, independent of other factors.[27]

The prevalence rates discussed previously are substantially higher than those reported from the previous NHANES data. Did the periodontal status of the United States get significantly worse in the intervening years? It is unlikely that this is the case. The most likely reason for the increase is that the methodology in the survey was changed based on input from an expert panel. Periodontal examination in older NHANES surveys consisted of partial mouth examinations, recording pocket depth, and gingival recession from only 2 sites per tooth and in teeth in only 2 quadrants of the mouth. In the most recent survey protocol, which began in 2009, full mouth examinations were conducted and pocket depth and gingival recession were measured on 6 sites per tooth. The result is that the new estimates of periodontal disease are far more accurate, whereas previous estimates most likely significantly under-reported the level of disease.[28]

ORAL CANCER

The American Cancer Society estimates that approximately 51,540 individuals will be diagnosed with oral cancer in 2018.[29] The rates of new cancers of the oral cavity and oropharynx, together commonly known as "oral cancer," have risen on average 0.6% each year over the past decade[30] and are the ninth most commonly diagnosed cancers in men (down from eighth in 2015). Reporting oral cancer rates as a combination of oral cavity and oropharyngeal cancers, however, masks the key fact that cancers of the oral cavity, which have as the major risk factors tobacco use and alcohol consumption, have been declining whereas oropharyngeal cancer incidence has been increasing.[31] Recently, human papillomavirus (HPV) infection has been recognized as a major risk factor for oropharyngeal cancer and is responsible for a portion of the increase in oropharyngeal cancer in White men and women. There are differences in outcomes between HPV-positive and HPV-negative oropharyngeal squamous cell cancer, with people having better survival outcomes if HPV-positive.[32] HPV-positive oropharyngeal cancers are more prevalent among White men and is expected to surpass the number of cervical cancers by 2020.[33,34] Despite that mortality rate for oral cancers overall has been decreasing over the past 3 decades and oral cancer is now ranked 14th in mortality rates, an estimated 10,030 people in the United States will die from these cancers in 2018.[29]

Oral cancers show marked age and gender disparities. Individuals aged 50 years to 69 years had a substantially higher risk for oropharyngeal cancer compared with cancers of the oral cavity. Individuals who were 70 years old or older had the highest overall oral cancer risk, and this risk was highest for cancers in the oral cavity.[31] Despite that the prevalence of oral cancer increases with age, more than 1 in 4 cases occur in patients younger than 55 years old.[29] There are also marked disparities based on gender, with men afflicted by oral cancer more than twice as often as women. Historically, Black men experienced the highest incidence of oral cancer. From 2000 to 2010, however, a break in this trend was documented and non-Hispanic White men had the highest age-adjusted incidence of oral and oropharyngeal cancer. During this decade, Black men experienced a decrease in both cancer of the oral cavity and oropharyngeal cancer, whereas White men showed an increase in oropharyngeal cancer. The latest data show that in men, oral cancers are approximately equally common in Blacks and in Whites, but Hispanics are still less likely to be affected. There is also some evidence that squamous cell carcinomas of the tongue are increasing in young, White women 18 years old to 44 years old, and little is known about the reason for this increase, but it seems unrelated to HPV.[35]

Although the incidence of oral cancer in Blacks and Whites has been similar in recent years, there are significant and persistent racial disparities in survival rates. The average 5-year survival for Blacks has been reported at 30% compared with 55% to 59% in Whites[36] Overall survival has been shown to be 40 months in Whites compared with 21 months in Blacks.[37] One contributing factor to this disparity is that Black patients tend to present with more advanced disease than White patients. One study found that 16% of Black men and 13% of Black women present with metastatic disease, compared with 9% and 8% in White men and women and that only 17% of African American men are diagnosed with localized disease compared with 32% of White men.[36]

Socioeconomic determinants of health have been assessed in the oral cancer populations to help explain the cause of this racial disparity. Gourin and Podolsey[38] found that African American patients lived in census block groups, with significantly lower mean education levels, median income, and a higher percentage of the population below the poverty line compared with White patients.[37,38] Poorer survival in African Americans was also associated with the traditional risk factors associated with poor oral cancer outcomes, such as alcohol abuse. The analysis showed racial disparity for insurance status; however, when socioeconomic factors, including insurance status, were controlled for in the analysis, the disparities in oral cancer outcomes were greatly diminished, although not eliminated.[36]

In summary, there has been a shift in the pattern of oral cancer. The overall rates have been slightly increasing for the past decade, but this information is not as clinically useful as if the disease patterns of the 2 distinct groups of cancers that comprise oral cancer were reported separately. Cancer of the oral cavity is declining, but older men, especially Black men, are at higher risk.[39] In younger women, cases of squamous cell carcinoma of the tongue are increasing. The primary risk factors for cancers of the oral cavity continue to be tobacco and alcohol use. Conversely, cancers of the oropharynx are increasing, largely driven by the increase in HPV-positive oropharyngeal cancer that are more often found in young, White men. These shifts have implications for changes in clinical practice, including risk assessment protocols, patient education, and medical/dental collaborations revolving around HPV vaccinations as a way to eliminate the rise in HPV related oral cancers.

OROFACIAL PAIN

According to the American Board of Orofacial Pain, "Orofacial pain is pain perceived in the face and/or oral cavity. It is caused by diseases or disorders of regional structures, by dysfunction of the nervous system, or through referral from distant sources" (**Box 1**).

Racial and ethnic disparities in regard to pain and its management have become increasingly recognized over the past 2 decades. For example, "racial and ethnic minorities tend to be undertreated for pain when compared with non-Hispanic Whites."[40] Work in the area of chronic orofacial pain and its management has also identified some important disparities. A major contribution to the field has been made by the National Institute of Dental and Craniofacial Research (NIDCR)-supported Orofacial Pain Prospective Evaluation and Risk Assessment (OPPERA) study. It has focused on TMD, a "heterogeneous family of musculoskeletal disorders that represent the most common chronic orofacial pain condition."[41] Prior to OPPERA, "most epidemiologic studies of TMD have been

---

Box 1
Scope of orofacial pain

The scope of orofacial pain includes diagnosis and treatment of but not limited to
- Intraoral, intracranial, extracranial, and systemic disorders that cause orofacial pain
- Complex masticatory and cervical musculoskeletal pain
- Neurovascular pain, that is, headache disorders resulting in orofacial pain
- Neuropathic pain
- Psychosocial concerns
- Sleep disorders related to orofacial pain
- Pain secondary to systemic disorders, such as cancer and AIDS
- Regional pain syndromes
- Orofacial movement disorders
- Other complex disorders causing persistent pain and dysfunction of the orofacial structures

From American Board of Orofacial Pain. What is orofacial pain? Available at: http://www.abop.net/?page=AboutOP. Accessed April 18, 2017; with permission.

limited to cross-sectional or case-control designs and have largely relied on convenience samples."[41] Recently, using OPPERA longitudinal data, Slade and colleagues[42] reported that "the rate of TMD symptoms in African Americans was twice that of Whites, and the rate of clinically verified TMD was 52% greater." This differed from earlier work using cross-sectional samples where TMD prevalence had been found consistently higher in non-Hispanic Whites. In the prospective study, the TMD incidence rate was not significantly different between men and women, different from findings in cross-sectional surveys. They explained their unexpected race and gender findings as due in part to prevalence-incidence bias that affects cross-sectional study designs. In the OPPERA case-control study, women were more likely than men and Whites more likely than African Americans to have persistent TMD 6 months after onset. This differential persistence makes prevalence more likely to be captured in a study measuring disease at only 1 time point.[42]

In contrast, and consistent with other work, Isong and colleagues[43] analyzed data from the 2002 NHIS and found that the prevalence of TMD and muscle disorder (TMJMD)-type pain was much lower in African Americans. Importantly, subsequent work by Plesh and colleagues,[44] using NHIS data from 2000 through 2005, found that the prevalence of TMJMD comorbid pains was much higher in Hispanics and non-Hispanic Blacks. For example, Hispanics and non-Hispanic Blacks reported more comorbid pain than non-Hispanic Whites (odds ratio [OR] = 1.56, $P<.001$; and OR = 1.38, $P<.001$, respectively). "In addition, 53% of those with TMJMD-type pain had severe headache/migraines; 54% had neck pain, 64% low back pain and 62% joint pain."[44] They conclude that to identify the underlying basis of these findings, it is important to "understand the role of psychosocial burden accumulated over the life span within socially disadvantaged groups to further address health disparities."

The Florida Dental Study[45] previously explored the role of socioeconomic and demographic disparities in orofacial pain symptoms. They found that adults over 45 years of age of lower socioeconomic status (SES) are at increased risk for orofacial pain and pain-related behavioral impact." In a study of 1636 community-north Floridians over 65 years of age, "racial differences were not found for 12-month prevalence or pain ratings for any painful oral symptom, or in the total number of symptoms. The most consistent racial differences were in behavioral impact associated with pain. Blacks reported greater behavioral impact as defined by pain having reduced their daily activities or motivating them to take some action in response to pain."[46] They concluded that "other pain-related variables, such as behavioral impacts, are useful when describing disparities associated with orofacial pain." A related factor is the important role that cultural beliefs and acculturation may play in understanding disparities, both in the psychosocial impacts and in the care of orofacial pain conditions. For example, in Hispanic adults "lower levels of acculturation, particularly less frequent use of English, were associated with greater oral pain and depression"[47] and decreased ability to access needed oral health care.

As Green and colleagues[40] noted, "the sources of pain disparities among racial and ethnic minorities are complex, involving patient (eg, patient/health care provider communication, attitudes), health care provider (eg, decision making), and health care system (eg, access to pain medication) factors." Pain arises from different underlying conditions with differences in individual levels of pain tolerance, willingness to admit pain, and pain-relief behaviors. Similar to medicine, there is a need in dentistry "for improved training for health care providers and educational interventions for patients."[40]

DISCUSSION

Most of the oral health disparities experienced in the United States and described in this article are avoidable and many argue are unjust because the disparities are largely experienced by those living in poverty and racial and ethnic minority groups. The US dental care system currently works well for those who can access high-quality and comprehensive care. Ironically, individuals who have the greatest access are those who often have the lowest risk for disease and need the care the least. Unfortunately, many low-income, low-educated, and disadvantaged populations with the highest levels of untreated dental disease are the very people who lack access to high-quality care for the multitude of reasons outlined in this article and described in detail in the Institute of Medicine report, *Unequal Treatment: Confronting Racial and Ethnic Disparities in Health Care*.[5] Importantly, many of these factors are under practitioners' control so there is hope that by working collaboratively as individual practitioners and through dental societies and other dental and health professional organizations, it is possible to bring an end to oral health disparities in the United States. Moving forward, dental education must continue to improve the Doctor of Dental Surgery/Doctor of Dental Medicine/Registered Dental Hygienist curriculum to ensure that the next generation of oral health professionals will (1) understand the epidemiology of health disparities; (2) have the awareness and skills to provide culturally sensitive treatment to diverse populations; (3) recognize and overcome the bias that they bring to clinical encounters with patients; (4) develop and implement effective strategies for bringing preventive care and treatment to those who currently have limited access; and (5) have the leadership skills to advocate for health policy changes that will improve the oral health of the entire population, not just their own patients. To ensure equitable access to high-quality care for the entire population, these practitioner level changes must be coupled with interventions at every other level of influence, including education of the public and changes in macro health policy that will improve the social determinants of health. This more upstream approach, however, is a more daunting undertaking and will require new innovative partnerships where dentistry is included in policy decisions that were previously seen as outside of that area of expertise. For example, participating in city planning, to ensure that neighborhoods are designed with access to affordable fresh fruits and vegetables and not just prepackaged foods that are higher in carbohydrates and more cariogenic, could have a significant positive impact on the oral health of those living within that region. Oral health professionals must also actively advocate for incorporation of oral health into new and existing health policy and form stronger alliances with the other health professions and health professional organizations.

As daunting as this may seem, within this article is an example of the tremendous success that such multilevel efforts can have on health disparities. Although the caries prevalence in children aged 2 years to 5 years remained stable over the past decade, the percentage of very young children with untreated decay has substantially decreased.[14] Although these findings have just been released and there has been no evidence that demonstrates this positive outcome is even partially attributable to the many initiatives aimed at this problem over the past 2 decades, it is a plausible hypothesis. The American Academy of Pediatric Dentistry advocated for children to have their first dental visit by age 1 and also formed strong alliances with the American Academy of Pediatrics, which in turn adopted this policy as a standard of pediatric practice,[48] thereby getting more young children enrolled in a dental home. NIDCR-supported oral health disparities research demonstrated the effectiveness of fluoride varnish in preventing dental caries in primary teeth of very young children.[49] This work provided the foundation for policy changes, such as

Medicaid reimbursement for fluoride varnish application by nondental health professionals. This change in reimbursement was instrumental in facilitating pediatric medical teams to provide fluoride varnish applications as well as oral health counseling, screenings, and referrals for dental visits for children beginning at age 1. These initiatives were coupled with parent outreach and media campaigns designed to change parental attitudes and increase demand for dental care for young children. This multipronged approach, which targeted patients, providers, the health care delivery and finance systems, and health policy changes, seems to have made an impact. Although success was achieved in getting children with disease into treatment, there was little change in caries prevalence in this age group so there is still work to be done in this area, particularly working with the medical field to find efficient strategies that will allow more oral health anticipatory guidance and greater uptake of fluoride varnish applications within pediatric practices. Another area of multilevel intervention that is gaining momentum is using lessons learned from tobacco cessation activities and applying those strategies to decrease sugar consumption in the United States. Because excess sugar consumption is a risk factor for many chronic diseases, it is an area that would naturally benefit from the combined expertise of many professions, including dentistry.

There are innumerable other opportunities for dentists and the dental profession to make an impact on oral health disparities. A long-standing opportunity is working on these same multiple levels of influence to decrease tobacco use in an effort to decrease risk for periodontal disease and oral cancers. Although screening for tobacco use and either providing the most current, evidence-based smoking cessation counseling in individual practices or referring for these services are important for individual patients, more can be done on a policy level and by partnering with other professions and professional organizations to collaboratively address this important public health issue. More recently, HPV infection also has been recognized as a major risk factor for oropharyngeal cancer. This has implications for changes in clinical practice, including risk assessment protocols, patient education, and medical/dental collaborations. If the dental profession takes an active role in defining, advocating for, and implementing these changes in concert with medical colleagues, it will improve long-term patient health outcomes.

Although the country has made strides to reduce some of the disparities originally described in *Oral Health in America: A Report of the Surgeon General*,[50] much work remains. Looking to the future, this is an exciting time for dentistry and there is the potential to make changes that significantly benefit the population as a whole, moving toward the elimination of the stark oral health disparities that persist. This is particularly important because as the US demographics are shifting toward increasing numbers of elders, Hispanics, and Blacks,[51] those same populations who currently experience greater levels of disease are more likely to experience oral health disparities. Individual dentists must work within practices and leverage the support of professional organizations and local community-based organizations and coalitions. Joining these groups, advocating for oral health and reduction of oral health disparities at meetings, and helping to connect key stakeholders on local and national levels are necessary steps forward that all can pledge to make. It will allow the profession to actively define the path forward instead of passively following the road set by others as the country struggles with the important issue of health disparities.

REFERENCES

1. Healthy People 2020. Washington, DC: U.S. Department of Health and Human Services, Office of Disease Prevention and Health Promotion. Available at:

https://www.healthypeople.gov/2020/about/foundation-health-measures/Disparities. Accessed April 15, 2017.

2. Whitehead M. The concepts and principles of equity and health. Int J Health Serv 1992;22(3):429–45.
3. Braveman P. What are health disparities and health equity? We need to be clear. Public Health Rep 2014;129(Suppl 2):5–8.
4. Braveman P. Health difference, disparity, inequality or inequity–what difference does it make what we cll it?. In: Buchbiner M, Rivkin-Fish M, Walker RL, editors. Understanding health inequalities and justice. Chapel Hill (NC): The University of North Carolina Press; 2016. p. 33–63.
5. Nelson A. Unequal treatment: confronting racial and ethnic disparities in health care. J Natl Med Assoc 2002;94(8):666–8.
6. U.S. Department of Health and Human Services. HHS action plan to reduce racial and ethnic health disparities. Washington, DC, 2011. Available at: https://minorityhealth.hhs.gov/npa/files/Plans/HHS/HHS_Plan_complete.pdf. Accessed April 15, 2017.
7. Ending racial and ethnic health disparities in the USA. Lancet 2011;377(9775):1379.
8. Satcher D, Nottingham JH. Revisiting oral health in america: a report of the surgeon general. Am J Public Health 2017;107(S1):S32–3.
9. Edelstein BL. The dental caries pandemic and disparities problem. BMC Oral Health 2006;6(Suppl 1):S2.
10. National Health and Nutrition Examination Survey. CDC/National Center for Health Statistics. Available at: https://www.cdc.gov/nchs/nhanes/index.htm. Accessed July 27, 2017.
11. National Cancer Institute. Surveillance, epidemiology, and end results program. Available at: https://seer.cancer.gov/. Accessed July 27, 2017.
12. National Health Interview Survey. CDC/National Center for Health Statistics. Available at: https://www.cdc.gov/nchs/nhis/index.htm. Accessed July 27, 2017.
13. Moeller J, Starkel R, Quinonez C, et al. Income inequality in the United States and its potential effect on oral health. J Am Dent Assoc 2017;148(6):361–8.
14. Dye BA, Mitnik GL, Iafolla TJ, et al. Trends in dental caries in children and adolescents according to poverty status in the United States from 1999 through 2004 and from 2011 through 2014. J Am Dent Assoc 2017;148(8):550–65.e7.
15. Healthy People 2020. Washington, DC: U.S. Department of Health and Human Services, Office of Disease Prevention and Health Promotion. Available at: https://www.healthypeople.gov/node/3511/data details. Accessed April 10, 2017.
16. Capurro DA, Iafolla T, Kingman A, et al. Trends in income-related inequality in untreated caries among children in the United States: findings from NHANES I, NHANES III, and NHANES 1999-2004. Community Dent Oral Epidemiol 2015;43(6):500–10.
17. Colby SL, Ortman JM. Projections of the size and composition of the U.S. population: 2014 to 2060. Washington, DC: U.S. Census Bureau; 2015. Available at: https://www.census.gov/content/dam/Census/library/publications/2015/demo/p25-1143.pdf.
18. Dye BA, Thornton-Evans G, Li X, et al. Dental caries and sealant prevalence in children and adolescents in the United States, 2011-2012. NCHS Data Brief 2015;(191):1–8.
19. Healthy People 2020. Washington, DC: U.S. Department of Health and Human Services, Office of Disease Prevention and Health Promotion. Available at: https://www.healthypeople.gov/2020/data/disparities/summary/Chart/5021/3. Accessed April 18, 2017.

20. Dye BA, Li X, Beltran-Aguilar ED. Selected oral health indicators in the United States, 2005-2008. NCHS Data Brief 2012;(96):1–8.

21. Wu B, Hybels C, Liang J, et al. Social stratification and tooth loss among middle-aged and older Americans from 1988 to 2004. Community Dent Oral Epidemiol 2014;42(6):495–502.

22. Dye B, Thornton-Evans G, Li X, et al. Dental caries and tooth loss in adults in the United States, 2011-2012. NCHS Data Brief 2015;(197):197.

23. National Health and Nutrition Examination Survey. Tooth loss in adults. Found at National Institute of Dental and Craniofacial Research. Available at: https://www.nidcr.nih.gov/DataStatistics/FindDataByTopic/ToothLoss/ToothLossAdults20to64.htm. Accessed April 17, 2017.

24. Healthy People 2020. Washington, DC: U.S. Department of Health and Human Services, Office of Disease Prevention and Health Promotion. Available at: https://www.healthypeople.gov/2020/data/disparities/summary/Chart/5025/5.1. Accessed April 19, 2017.

25. Eke PI, Page RC, Wei L, et al. Update of the case definitions for population-based surveillance of periodontitis. J Periodontol 2012;83(12):1449–54.

26. Eke PI, Wei L, Thornton-Evans GO, et al. Risk indicators for periodontitis in US adults: NHANES 2009 to 2012. J Periodontol 2016;87(10):1174–85.

27. Eke PI, Dye BA, Wei L, et al, CDC Periodontal Disease Surveillance workgroup: James Beck (University of North Carolina, Chapel Hill, USA), Gordon Douglass (Past President, American Academy of Periodontology), Roy Page (University of Washin. Prevalence of periodontitis in adults in the United States: 2009 and 2010. J Dent Res 2012;91(10):914–20.

28. Eke PI. Self-reported current or prior periodontal disease performs moderately well in characterizing periodontitis status in postmenopausal women who receive regular dental checkups. J Evid Based Dent Pract 2015;15(3):121–3.

29. American Cancer Society. About oral cavity and oropharyngeal cancer. Available at: https://www.cancer.org/cancer/oral-cavity-and-oropharyngeal-cancer/about/key-statistics.html. Accessed April 15, 2017.

30. National Cancer Institute. Surveillance, epidemiology, and end results program. Available at: https://seer.cancer.gov/statfacts/html/oralcav.html. Accessed July 26, 2017.

31. Weatherspoon DJ, Chattopadhyay A, Boroumand S, et al. Oral cavity and oropharyngeal cancer incidence trends and disparities in the United States: 2000-2010. Cancer Epidemiol 2015;39(4):497–504.

32. Dalianis T. Human papillomavirus and oropharyngeal cancer, the epidemics, and significance of additional clinical biomarkers for prediction of response to therapy (Review). Int J Oncol 2014;44(6):1799–805.

33. Chaturvedi AK, Engels EA, Pfeiffer RM, et al. Human papillomavirus and rising oropharyngeal cancer incidence in the United States. J Clin Oncol 2011;29(32):4294–301.

34. Cleveland JL, Junger ML, Saraiya M, et al. The connection between human papillomavirus and oropharyngeal squamous cell carcinomas in the United States: implications for dentistry. J Am Dent Assoc 2011;142(8):915–24.

35. Patel SC, Carpenter WR, Tyree S, et al. Increasing incidence of oral tongue squamous cell carcinoma in young white women, age 18 to 44 years. J Clin Oncol 2011;29(11):1488–94.

36. Goodwin WJ, Thomas GR, Parker DF, et al. Unequal burden of head and neck cancer in the United States. Head Neck 2008;30(3):358–71.

37. Molina MA, Cheung MC, Perez EA, et al. African American and poor patients have a dramatically worse prognosis for head and neck cancer: an examination of 20,915 patients. Cancer 2008;113(10):2797–806.
38. Gourin CG, Podolsky RH. Racial disparities in patients with head and neck squamous cell carcinoma. Laryngoscope 2006;116(7):1093–106.
39. LeHew CW, Weatherspoon DJ, Peterson CE, et al. The health system and policy implications of changing epidemiology for oral cavity and oropharyngeal cancers in the United States from 1995 to 2016. Epidemiol Rev 2017;39(1):132–47.
40. Green CR, Anderson KO, Baker TA, et al. The unequal burden of pain: confronting racial and ethnic disparities in pain. Pain Med 2003;4(3):277–94.
41. Maixner W, Diatchenko L, Dubner R, et al. Orofacial pain prospective evaluation and risk assessment study–the OPPERA study. J Pain 2011;12(11 Suppl): T4–11.e1-2.
42. Slade GD, Ohrbach R, Greenspan JD, et al. Painful temporomandibular disorder: decade of discovery from OPPERA studies. J Dent Res 2016;95(10):1084–92.
43. Isong U, Gansky SA, Plesh O. Temporomandibular joint and muscle disorder-type pain in U.S. adults: the national health interview survey. J Orofac Pain 2008;22(4): 317–22.
44. Plesh O, Adams SH, Gansky SA. Temporomandibular joint and muscle disorder-type pain and comorbid pains in a national US sample. J Orofac Pain 2011;25(3): 190–8.
45. Riley JL 3rd, Gilbert GH, Heft MW. Socioeconomic and demographic disparities in symptoms of orofacial pain. J Public Health Dent 2003;63(3):166–73.
46. Riley JL 3rd, Gilbert GH, Heft MW. Orofacial pain: racial and sex differences among older adults. J Public Health Dent 2002;62(3):132–9.
47. Riley JL 3rd, Gibson E, Zsembik BA, et al. Acculturation and orofacial pain among Hispanic adults. J Pain 2008;9(8):750–8.
48. Section On Oral Health. Maintaining and improving the oral health of young children. Pediatrics 2014;134(6):1224–9.
49. Weintraub JA, Ramos-Gomez F, Jue B, et al. Fluoride varnish efficacy in preventing early childhood caries. J Dent Res 2006;85(2):172–6.
50. US Department of Health and Human Services. Oral Health in America: A Report of the Surgeon General – Executive Summary. Rockville, MD: US Department of Health and Human Services, National Institute of Dental and Craniofacial Research, National Institutes of Health 2000.
51. Vincent GK, Velkoff VA. The next four decades, the older population in the United States: 2010 to 2050, current population reports, P25–1138. Washington, DC: U.S. Census Bureau; 2010.

The Expanding Dental Workforce
The Impact of Nondental Providers

Hugh Silk, MD, MPH

KEYWORDS

- Oral health • Health education • Interprofessional relations • Dental education

KEY POINTS

- National medical institutions (eg, Institute of Medicine, Healthy People 2020, and so forth) have made oral health a priority for addressing overall health over the past decade.
- Health professional and educational organizations from family medicine to midwifery are evolving to challenge their learners and clinicians to address oral health.
- Specific efforts from groups like the National Interprofessional Initiative on Oral Health and Qualis Health are implementing practical education and office-based strategies.
- Ultimately, interprofessional efforts with a focus on patient outcomes (and not professional turf boundaries) will result in the best overall results.
- Future efforts will take a massive centrally organized effort of many governmental and nongovernmental agencies, academies, and associations.

THE EVOLUTION OF NONDENTAL HEALTH PROVIDERS ENGAGING IN ORAL HEALTH

Medical providers are taught to care for whole patients within the context of their social and community parameters. As part of this broad approach to addressing wellness, most health fields have begun to embrace the importance of oral health. These efforts began with the surgeon general's report on oral health in 2000.[1] This pivotal moment caused health professions to take note of the impact of oral health on overall health. David Satcher made it clear that nondental health professionals had not only a role but also a responsibility. This statement led to the 2003 *National Call to Action to Promote Oral Health* document[2] defining the importance of oral health and the pathway to more interprofessional collaboration.

At the same time, the American Academy of Pediatrics (AAP) formed the Section on Oral Health to help facilitate the AAP membership becoming more aware of oral health

Disclosure Statement: The author has nothing to declare.
Department of Family Medicine and Community Health, University of Massachusetts Medical School, Community Healthlink, 40 Spruce Street, Leominster, MA 01453, USA
E-mail address: hugh.silk@umassmed.edu

Dent Clin N Am 62 (2018) 195–206
https://doi.org/10.1016/j.cden.2017.11.002
0011-8532/18/© 2017 Elsevier Inc. All rights reserved.

dental.theclinics.com

issues.[3] Over time the AAP developed a comprehensive curriculum entitled Protecting All Children's Tooth[4] among other initiatives. This curriculum was followed by the Society of Teachers in Family Medicine (2003) creating the Group on Oral Health. This initiative led to the creation of a national curriculum for health providers entitled Smiles for Life (which has since been used by more than 1000000 medical and dental professionals).[5] These initiatives had an influence on the creation of oral health residency requirements and board examination questions in family medicine and pediatrics.

A surge of efforts occurred in 2010 and 2011 with respect to the entire health force becoming engaged in oral health. It began with the Health and Human Services (HHS) creating the Oral Health Initiative (2010).[6] This initiative reinforced the idea that oral health was within the realm of all health care. At the same time, the National Interprofessional Initiative on Oral Health (NIIOH) was formed through foundational support (DentaQuest Foundation, Washington Dental Health Foundation, Connecticut Health Foundation, and later the REACH Healthcare Foundation).[7] The NIIOH focused on health training programs and stimulated specialties like physician assistants, nursing, pharmacy and midwifery to engage in oral health.

In 2011, the Institute of Medicine (IOM) published *Advancing Oral Health in America*.[8] This landmark document assessed the state of oral health in the nondental professions, including nursing, obstetrics, and pharmacy. A companion document from the IOM, *Improving Access to Oral Health Care for Vulnerable and Underserved Populations*, assessed educational settings and challenged professions like social work and internal medicine to do more.[9] These initiatives led many professions to define core oral health competencies and evaluation tools for their specialty.

Both nursing and physician assistants held national summits and engaged the leadership of multiple national organizations about the importance of oral health and what their professions could do specifically. These summits stimulated new curricula, a series of articles in peer-reviewed journals, and changes on board examinations and program requirements.[10,11] Medical schools were also engaged during this period. The American Association of Medical Colleges (AAMC), with funding from the Health Resources and Services Administration (HRSA), created core oral health competencies for medical schools. These competencies were coupled with an enhancement of oral health curricula added to MedEdPORTAL (the AAMC's curricula repository) making practical oral health modules and resources readily available.[12]

Health education during this time was also embracing the concept of interprofessional education (IPE) and interprofessional practice (IPP). Oral health quickly became a logical topic to achieve such educational experience. The American Dental Education Association (ADEA) teamed up with 5 other influential health education organizations (including nursing, pharmacy, public health, and osteopathic and allopathic medicine) to create core competencies for IPE and IPP. This collaboration became a catalyst for health and dental schools to work together on cases and in clinical settings to learn about team care.[13]

Meanwhile, Healthy People 2020 included oral health markers as one of the top 9 leading health indicators.[14] This inclusion sent a message to health providers that they too would be held accountable for oral health public health measures.

Efforts at the educational level, and public health level, were followed by changes at a clinical level. Medicaid began this effort by reimbursing medical offices for oral health evaluations and application of fluoride varnish for children (which included all 50 states by 2017). State-wide efforts trained medical staff and helped them evolve office flow, and oral health prompts were added to electronic health records (EHRs). With the signing of the Affordable Care Act (ACA) and its emphasis on prevention, oral health was soon solidified into the medical realm. The ACA mandated that all US Preventive Services Task Force (USPSTF) level A and B recommendations be covered by all insurers. In 2014, the application of fluoride varnish by medical providers for those younger than 6 years became a level B recommendation, which led to a dramatic increase in oral health screens and fluoride varnish application in primary care offices.[15–17]

ORAL HEALTH IS A NATURAL FIT WITHIN HEALTH CARE

Oral disease is a chronic illness that requires prevention, screening, early detection, management, and reevaluation. The medical model is based on a patient-centered, preventive, chronic management approach and is in the process of getting health providers to also think about their patients on a population level. This approach is how medicine already deals with everything from breast cancer to diabetes, so it only makes sense for medical and health professionals to be playing a more active role in oral health care.

The traditional oral health system has a lack of capacity. Although some of this is related to a lack of dentists in certain parts of the country, it also involves dental care not being available where people spend their time: schools, community centers, homes, and so forth. If we think of the health team in its broadest sense, everyone engages with a health professional on most days. Children are in schools engaging with school nurses and school-health clinics; many people have contact with social workers; most patients visit the pharmacy for medications and health advice. More formally, there are more than 550 million visits to primary care providers (PCPs) annually.[18] However, most of the population does not visit a dentist in any given year; the goal for annual dental visits for Healthy People 2020 remains at less than 50%.[19] So although many people are engaging with numerous health professionals, they are not always seeing a dental provider.

Health care providers are used to caring for the underserved. The health care system uses creative means to provide care outside of traditional health centers. The elderly are seen in nursing homes; the homeless are seen by mobile care units; and rural dwellers are seen via home care. Primary care providers, social workers, and community health workers know their patients well and understand the barriers patients face. It is not a stretch to have them add oral health care to their current regimen.

Many health care providers are used to expanding their scope of care. They learn new techniques, skills, and approaches to meet the needs of patients. For example, a family doctor practicing in an area where there is a shortage of gynecologists will learn how to perform colposcopy or how to inject joints where there are not enough orthopedists. In the oral health realm, pediatric providers have embraced learning how to apply fluoride varnish to address the gap of young children receiving this service in the dental setting.

Many areas of medicine directly affect the mouth, so it is impractical to think the field would not address oral health. For example, physicians and pharmacists oversee a massive disbursement of medications, many of which effect the mouth (eg, xerostomia, candidiasis, and so forth). The health care team is facing unprecedented levels of substance abuse (eg, tobacco, alcohol, opioids), which has a direct effect on oral pathologic conditions such as oral cancers. Lastly, many inflammatory conditions (eg, diabetes, rheumatoid arthritis) have an intricate relationship of mouth and body, especially with periodontitis. Studies have shown that those with diabetes, for example, that address their periodontitis have lower health care costs and hospitalizations.[20] Furthermore, oral caries can affect one's confidence and social well-being, which is certainly in the domain of the health practitioner.[21]

Health care students are being taught the importance of team care through IPE, and providers are being challenged to embrace IPP. Current examples of oral health being included in IPE include physical therapists at the Bouvé College of Health Sciences at Northeastern University doing oral health screenings and medical students learning in the dental clinic at Virginia Tech Carilion School of Medicine.[22,23] Some nursing teams are already integrating with dental providers in a comprehensive clinical model (eg, New York University's schools of nursing and dentistry).[24]

The patient-centered medical home is the current approach to creating coordinated, comprehensive, and accessible care. Qualis Health has made it a priority for oral health to have a key role in medical homes.[25] Qualis Health has provided PCPs with tools for systems change to ensure that oral care and referrals are embedded in office visits. Examples of this integration include Wenatchee Clinic's Pediatric Department (Washington) providing routine oral health evaluations and fluoride varnish for all children/adolescents. At the Marshfield clinic (Wisconsin), searches are done in the EHR to assess if diabetic patients have had recent routine dental visits; if not, they are contacted to make appointments.[26]

CURRENT TRENDS IN ORAL HEALTH EDUCATION AND PRACTICE IN THE HEALTH PROFESSIONS

There is a current convergence of efforts that is driving oral health into the mainstream of primary care. The DentaQuest Foundation has been supporting projects for years to create better medical-dental integration. They now have a 50-state approach organized into regional efforts. Each state and region is charged with advancing the DentaQuest 2020 goals that span creating a Medicare oral health benefit to improving oral health access within schools. DentaQuest has been a supporter of Smiles for Life since its inception (the national interprofessional oral health curriculum designed for all health professions to learn basic oral health concepts on topics across the life span). DentaQuest has funded projects in many states that have trained medical offices and health schools to address pediatric oral health and offer fluoride varnish to children.

Meanwhile, government-based efforts have synergized these efforts. In 2014, the HRSA published the white paper on "Integration of Oral Health and Primary Care Practice."[27] This document focused on the role of primary care in administering oral health services. This document was soon followed with another white paper from Qualis Health entitled "Oral Health: An Essential Component of Primary Care."[26] Qualis recently published a companion document with more details based on a series of trials of their previously proposed interventions.[28] The focus of these white papers was to offer very concrete examples for busy PCPs to work oral health screening, management, and referrals into their already taxed system of seeing patients. The documents include examples from across the country that have been effective and flow diagrams to think about a role for each team member, thus, reducing the burden of effort on any one person in a medical office. For example, the nurse can ask about recent fluoride varnish use and apply the varnish; the medical assistant can make a dental referral; and the PCP can do the oral examination and offer dental hygiene advice.

Although primary care has been the focus of many oral health integration efforts, others have chosen to think about a broader approach. Again, HRSA has awarded grants to states to engage obstetric providers to ask about and address oral health through advice and referrals. These efforts are based on the premise that if a mother has better oral health and hygiene habits and a regular dental home, then her child is much more likely to have the same. These projects have been training dentists, midwives, obstetricians, family physicians, and others to have common messaging and approaches to addressing oral health in prenatal patients.

The NIIOH has also been inclusive in their efforts working with medical and dental professionals to increase efforts on an educational level originally and more recently in the clinical realm as well. The NIIOH has annually brought together leaders from traditional as well as nontraditional fields, including pharmacy, community health care workers, and medical assistants, to encourage them to add oral health to their professional training. This effort has resulted in many health specialties adding oral health curriculum locally and nationally under the influences of the NIIOH, ADEA, and others.[29,30]

NEXT STEPS: A COMPREHENSIVE NATIONAL APPROACH TO ORAL HEALTH AND HEALTH

Oral health includes many dimensions. It starts with an understanding of the oral-systemic connection. It continues with addressing topics across the life span from caries and trauma to energy drink consumption and oral piercings. Oral disease has preventive, urgent, and chronic components as well as biopsychosocial, environmental, and socioeconomic implications. Health schools need a comprehensive oral health curriculum woven into mainstream topics and ideally offered with an interprofessional team approach.

There is a long way to go to achieve this goal. Even though some schools and professions have embraced oral health education and practice, many have not. Surveys of medical schools show that only 30.0% report having an oral health component, with 59.1% of these schools providing between 1 and 4 hours of oral health education over 4 years.[31] Nearly two-thirds of the surveyed pediatricians and family physicians report never receiving oral health education during their predoctoral training, and nearly half indicate a lack of continuing education in oral health following residency programs.[32] Obstetric training is even worse, with only 39% of residency programs having prenatal oral health training.[33]

But there is hope. Physician assistants are teaching oral health in almost 80% of their programs across the country.[34] In a recent survey of midwives, more than 90% reported explaining the role of early childhood caries to mothers and 80% were addressing the importance of dental visits for small children.[35] Several medical schools are also offering robust oral health curricula. The University of Massachusetts Medical School, for example, offers a spiral oral health curriculum covering topics from anatomy to population health.[36] And Virginia Tech Carilion School of Medicine has a week-long experience in oral health for all students and an endowed oral health curriculum.[23]

In the future, all levels of health education will need to require core oral health and IPE competencies. Many organizations already have these (AAMC, Physician Assistant Education Association [PAEA], HRSA).[13,37,38] The competencies should be included in accreditation standards to give them more influence. Oral health requirements for specialties, such as family medicine and pediatrics residencies, were removed to simplify standards. The Residency Review Committee should reinstall the oral health requirements.

Evaluation of oral health curricula is significantly lacking. Fewer than one-third of medical schools, for example, have any form of assessment.[31] Evaluation needs to be clinically based and practical. Programs should borrow from those who have strong tools in place. Health profession schools, such as the Boston University Physician Assistant Program, are using standardized patients, objective structured clinical examinations, case reviews, and clinical exposures.[66] These experiences should be replicated with a diversity of patient populations and ages as well as in a variety of settings.

Educational changes will help the next generation of doctors, nurses, and physician assistants; however, we also need improvements in clinical practice in order to have more immediate results. Medicine will have to intervene across all medical/health settings, including office, hospital, emergency, and urgent care settings. Currently, 1% to 2% of all emergency department (ED) visits are for oral health issues.[40] This will require a better ED diversion approach so that patients are triaged and connected to dental care. Efforts are underway in several states to bridge this medical-dental gap.[41]

Some states have had tremendous success with getting PCPs to address pediatric oral health. North Carolina has championed this effort for years and proven that physicians can identify the presence of dental disease, apply fluoride varnish, and lower rates of caries.[42,43] Other efforts are simplifying and validating how nondental professionals can perform concise and accurate oral health risk assessments.[44] These efforts need to be expanded to all 50 states and territories and evolve to include programs aimed at adults, seniors, and other vulnerable populations (eg, homeless, prisoners) as evidence evolves.

We continue to underutilize oral health promotion and management in settings where the public engages with nontraditional health providers (eg, community centers, at home, and in long-term care facilities). Other nonconventional settings have already ramped up oral health promotion: Head Start; Women, Infants, and Children; and school health centers. Medical and allied health professionals could extend care through the use of tele-dentistry to reach the underserved. This practice is already happening in New York.[45] Practical training and consults can also occur through initiatives, such as Project ECHO (currently training PCPs to directly treat conditions like hepatitis C).[46]

Another format for extending health care to those in need is for dental professionals to be present in medical settings and vice versa. Blurring the lines of professional parameters in a disruptive manner can produce results exponentially faster than tweaking existing systems. Referrals are improved with warm handoffs whereby patients are introduced to dental team members to improve adherence (eg, Arizona Alliance for Community Health Centers and Safety Net Solutions).[47,48] Taking this to another level includes dental professionals offering care outside of their traditional setting. For example, in New Hampshire, one dental hygienist currently sees prenatal patients in the obstetrics/gynecology office and triages them to the dental setting as needed.[49]

Conversely, medical providers are integrating medical care into dental settings. HRSA is already investing in this model; at the Harvard School of Dental Medicine, nurse practitioners offer primary care within the dental setting.[50] Even without medical providers being present in dental settings, studies show that dentists, physicians, and patients are all comfortable with dental providers offering medical screenings (eg, blood pressure).[51–53] With so many people lapsing on medical care, screening in other settings makes sense.

For real change to occur, both rewards and penalties for providers to address oral health will be needed. For example, some medical boards have added oral health questions on their examinations (eg, family medicine, pediatrics).[54] All relevant health professions need to replicate this. EHRs are and should continue to evolve oral health prompts to ensure the systematic offering of oral hygiene advice, screening, and effective referrals. This offering must be coupled with a sharing of health information in real time. A shared EHR is currently being used in the Marshfield clinic (Wisconsin).[55] This sharing allows the health system to search all patients with diabetes, for example, to see if they have had dental care. Systems could be set up to see if patients are up to date on health screens in a dental setting and likewise dental screenings during a medical appointment. In areas where EHRs cannot be shared, a better cloud system could be used.

Efforts focused on medical and other health professions will not be enough if they are not done in a team manner. Health care already uses IPP for many diseases, such as diabetes and heart disease. Medical teams should be creative in adding newer team members to address oral health, such as dental hygienists, community health workers, and health coaches. Pilot projects are already showing positive effects in Federally Qualified Health Centers, improving medical-dental integration for patients with diabetes and pregnancy (eg, Harborview Medical Center, Seattle, Washington).[28]

Real change will come as health finances include medical-dental integration. Early observational studies have shown that patients with diabetes and strokes have reduced costs and fewer hospitalizations when they receive dental care compared with those who do not.[20] Accountable Care Organizations (ACOs) have picked up on this and are reducing overall health costs by including dental care within medical insurance (eg, Hennepin Health, Minnesota).[56]

Education and practice changes will have a dramatic impact on oral health for the population. These efforts are essential and yet need to be supported by larger public health efforts that have a foundation in the medical community. Medical health care professionals are well-respected members within their community. They can impact issues like water fluoridation and mouth-guard campaigns. In Massachusetts, the Massachusetts Medical Society has a committee on oral health whereby physicians and dentists work together on important oral health issues.[57] Health professional organizations should promote oral health messages to their membership and to the public. This promotion requires interprofessional/multispecialty committees, such as the Section on Oral Health within the AAP.[3]

HOW TO GET TO THE FUTURE: THE DIFFICULT ROAD AHEAD

Both medical and dental professionals have to embrace the idea that all health team members will have new roles and responsibilities. The way forward will not be easy. At the same time, it has already begun. This process began with IPE, IPP, and ACOs. Medical and dental care is already changing rapidly. Patients are demanding care in different settings (eg, urgent care, minute clinics) and by new types of professionals (allied health, dental therapists). Many traditionalists will challenge these changes and try to put the genie back in the bottle. These efforts to preserve the old system may slow progress but will not prevent it. Patients vote with their feet. HRSA, Qualis, the AAP, and others are already on board and helping providers to change their practice. The ultimate goal has to be better patient and population outcomes, not simply less disease but, rather, more oral health wellness.

Likely this will take learning powerful lessons in smaller settings (eg, local projects and modeling) and promoting them to a national audience. Creative ideas need to be collected and shared in a coordinated manner to got them to scale using social media and other technology (eg, webinars).

Improved oral health outcomes will require specialties to forego turf wars and allow boundaries of care to be expanded. Practice regulations will have to be adjusted. Medical and dental organizations will have to work more closely together. This collaboration will require more oral health interest groups and interprofessional committees. Current examples include the American Academy of Family Physicians' (AAFP's) Oral Health Member Interest Group and the American Dental Association's (ADA's) Committee on Access, Prevention, and Interprofessional Relations.[58]

There are many tools that could be used in nontraditional dental settings with the proper training. PCPs are used to learning a range of office-based procedures (eg, skin surgery, joint injections).[59] Alternative restorative treatments and silver diamine fluoride could be taught and implemented in areas lacking dentists. There are already physicians in one rural area (Maine) who perform extractions because of a dental shortage.[60] It is not practical to have all PCPs learn skills such as extractions; however, for some unique areas this may be the only choice. Health care teams could easily be taught to medically manage periodontitis with antibiotics (as an alternative or adjunct to deep root scaling). Currently, sealants are underutilized. Medical offices or school-based clinics could provide this service with proper training and equipment.

These changes are bold. And they will require bold individuals and organizations to champion and manage them. State and national health societies/academies could require continuing education in oral health. This should start with on-line courses and annual meeting presentations. Many organizations (AAFP, AAP, PAEA) are already providing such courses.

Currently, some health professionals must complete a quality improvement project when recertifying their board certification. Oral health is an option being offered to family physicians and pediatricians (eg, AAP, Education in Quality Improvement for Pediatric Practice modules).[61] More professions could do the same.

Medicine is trying to improve quality through the establishment of quality metrics. Oral health is already being considered for quality markers (eg, Vermont, fluoride varnish; Massachusetts Medicaid ACO, dental referrals). More systems will have to include oral health across the life span in quality metrics for this to have a significant impact. Likewise, reimbursement reform will have to continue and honor real outcomes, such as fewer caries, higher patient satisfaction, and hard-to-measure results like oral health wellness.

A well-orchestrated health system that includes meaningful oral health will take a massive, well-coordinated effort by influential national organizations. The IOM's Advance of Oral Health in America document called for an "oral health initiative leader." This leadership department would be housed in the HHS. It would require working with many other departments and organizations: the Centers for Medicare and Medicaid Services; USPSTF; Early and Periodic Screening, Diagnosis and Treatment; Centers for Disease Control and Prevention; Bureau of Primary Health Care; Bureau of Health Professions; Maternal and Child Health Bureau; National Institutes of Health; Indian Health Service; HRSA; Department of Education; and medical/dental organizations, such as the ADA, American Medical Association, American Physician Assistant Association, American Nurses Association, AAMC, ADEA, and others.

These broad changes will require interest from many organizations that may have had little interest in oral health heretofore. It will require societal change whereby the public is educated to understand the important role of the oral-systemic connection. Concepts such as "the mouth as part of the body" and "wellness as more than the absence of disease" need to be embraced going forward. This change is doable with the right leadership, effort level, and financial backing.

REFERENCES

1. U.S. Department of Health and Human. Oral health in America: a report of the surgeon general. Rockville (MD): U.S. Department of Health and Human Services, National Institute of Dental and Craniofacial Research, National Institutes of Health; 2000.

2. U.S. Department of Health and Human Services. A national call to action to promote oral health. Rockville (MD): U.S. Department of Health and Human Services, Public Health Service, Centers for Disease Control and Prevention, National Institutes of Health, National Institute of Dental and Craniofacial Research. NIH Publication No. 03-5303; 2003.
3. American Academy of Pediatrics section on oral health. Available at: https://www.aap.org/en-us/about-the-aap/Committees-Councils-Sections/Membership-Criteria/Pages/Oral-Health.aspx. Accessed May 14, 2017.
4. American Academy of Pediatrics. Protecting all children's teeth: a pediatric oral health training program. Available at: https://www.aap.org/en-us/advocacy-and-policy/aap-health-initiatives/Oral-Health/Pages/Education-and-Training.aspx. Accessed May 14, 2017.
5. Clark MB, Douglass AB, Maier R, et al. Smiles for life: a national oral health curriculum. 3rd edition. Society of Teachers of Family Medicine; 2010. Available at: www.smilesforlifeoralhealth.com. Accessed May 14, 2017.
6. Health and Human Services Oral Health Initiative 2010. Available at: http://www.hrsa.gov/publichealth/clinical/oralhealth/. Accessed May 14, 2017.
7. National Interprofessional Initiative on Oral Health. Available at: http://www.niioh.org/Accessed May 14, 2017.
8. IOM (Institute of Medicine). Advancing oral health in America. Washington, DC: The National Academies Press; 2011.
9. IOM (Institute of Medicine) and NRC (National Research Council). Improving access to oral health care for vulnerable and underserved populations. Washington, DC: The National Academies Press; 2011.
10. NYU College of Nursing. Oral health nursing education and practice. Available at: http://www.ohnep.org/. Accessed May 14, 2017.
11. American Academy of Physician Assistants. Oral health initiative. Available at: https://www.aapa.org/oralhealth/. Accessed May 14, 2017.
12. Association of American Medical Colleges. Oral health in medicine model curriculum. Available at: https://www.mededportal.org/collections/oralhealth/. Accessed May 14, 2017.
13. Interprofessional Education Collaborative Expert Panel. Core competencies for interprofessional collaborative practice: report of an expert panel. Washington, DC: Interprofessional Education Collaborative; 2011. Available at: https://www.aamc.org/download/186750/data/core_competencies.pdf. Accessed May 14, 2017.
14. Healthy People 2020. Oral health. Available at: http://www.healthypeople.gov/2020/topics-objectives/topic/oral-health. Accessed May 14, 2017.
15. United States Preventive Services Task Force. Dental caries in children birth through five years. 2014. Available at: http://www.uspreventiveservicestaskforce.org/Page/Document/UpdateSummaryFinal/dental-caries-in-children-from-birth-through-age-5-years-screening. Accessed May 14, 2017.
16. Okunseri C, Szabo A, Jackson S, et al. Increased children's access to fluoride varnish treatment by involving medical care providers: effect of a Medicaid policy change. Health Serv Res 2009;44(4):1144–56.
17. Dooley D, Moultrie NM, Heckman B, et al. Oral health prevention and toddler well-child care: routine integration in a safety net system. Pediatrics 2016;137(1):e40143532.
18. National Ambulatory Medical Care Survey: 2010 summary table. Available at: http://www.cdc.gov/nchs/data/ahcd/namcs_summary/2010_namcs_web_tables.pdf. Accessed May 14, 2017.

19. Healthy People 2020. Dental visits in the past twelve months, 2000. Available at http://www.healthypeople.gov/2020/leading-health-indicators/infographic/oral-health-2?width=618&height=100%25&date=Aug-2012. Accessed May 14, 2017.

20. Jeffcoat MK, Jeffcoat RL, Gladkowski PA, et al. Impact of periodontal therapy on general health: evidence from insurance data for five systemic conditions. Am J Prev Med 2014;47(2):166–74.

21. Guarnizo-Herreño CC, Wehby GL. Children's dental health, school performance and psychosocial well-being. J Pediatr 2012;161(6):1153–9.e2.

22. Northeastern University Bouve College of Health Sciences. Physical therapists promote oral health care. Innovations in oral health. Available at: http://www.northeastern.edu/oralhealth/physical-therapists-promote-oral-health-care/. Accessed May 14, 2017.

23. Virginia Tech Carilion School of Medicine and Research Institute. Oral health program. Available at: http://medicine.vtc.vt.edu/education/oral_health_program/. Accessed May 14, 2017.

24. Examples of the NYU College of Dentistry/NYU College of Nursing Alliance. Available at: http://dental.nyu.edu/aboutus/interprofessional-education.html. Accessed May 14, 2017.

25. Qualis Health. Oral health integration in the patient-centered medical home (PCMH) environment. Case studies from community health centers. 2012. Available at: http://www.qualishealth.org/sites/default/files/white-paper-oral-health-integration-pcmh.pdf. Accessed May 14, 2017.

26. Qualis Health. Oral health: an essential component of primary care. Case examples. June 2015. Available at: http://www.niioh.org/sites/default/files/Oral_Health_white_paper_case_examples.pdf. Accessed May 14, 2017.

27. US Department of Health and Human Services. Health resources and services administration. Integration of oral health and primary care practice. Feb 2014. Available at: http://www.hrsa.gov/publichealth/clinical/oralhealth/primarycare/integrationoforalhealth.pdf. Accessed May 14, 2017.

28. Hummel J, Phillips KA, Holt B, et al. Safety net medical home initiative. Organized, evidence-based care supplement: oral health integration. Seattle (WA): Qualis; 2016. Available at: http://practicetransformation.qualishealth.org/sites/default/files/practicetransformation.qualishealth.org/Executive-Summary-Oral-Health-Integration.pdf. Accessed May 14, 2017.

29. PAEA Receives Second Oral Health Grant. Available at: http://paeaonline.org/alerts/paea-receives-second-oral-health-grant/. Accessed May 14, 2017.

30. NYU Nursing's Oral Health Nursing Education and Practice (OHNEP) program launches Interprofessional Oral Health Faculty Toolkit. Available at: https://www.nyu.edu/about/news-publications/news/2015/march/nyu-nursings-oral-health-nursing-education-and-practice-ohnep-program-launches-interprofessional-oral-health-faculty-toolkit.html. Accessed May 14, 2017.

31. Ferullo A, Silk H, Savageau JA. Teaching oral health in U.S. medical schools: results of a national survey. Acad Med 2011;86(2):226–30.

32. Krol DM. Educating pediatricians on children's oral health: past, present, and future. Pediatrics 2004;113(5):e487–92.

33. Curtis M, Silk H, Savageau J. Prenatal oral health education in U.S. dental schools and obstetrics and gynecology residencies. J Dental Education 2013;77(11):1461–8.

34. Langelier MH, Glicken AD, Surdu S. Adoption of oral health curriculum by physician assistant education programs in 2014. J Physician Assist Educ 2015;26(2):60–9.

35. Ehlers V, Callaway A, Azrak B, et al. Survey of midwives' knowledge of caries prevention in perinatal care. MCN Am J Matern Child Nurs 2014;39(4):253–9.

36. University of Massachusetts Medical School. Oral health "spiral" curriculum. Available at: http://www.umassmed.edu/globalassets/family-medicine-and-community-health/fmch-community-health/documents/microsoft-word---aa-umms-oral-health-spiral-curriculum.pdf. Accessed May 14, 2017.

37. Association of American Medical Colleges. Oral health in medicine for the undergraduate medical education curriculum 2008. Available at: https://www.mededportal.org/download/306716/data/oralhealthinmedicinecomprehensions.pdf. Accessed May 14, 2017.

38. Danielsen R, Dillenberg J, Bay C. Oral health competencies for physician assistants and nurse practitioners. J Physician Assist Educ 2006;17(4):12–6.

39. Berkowitz OL, Kaufman LB, Russell M. Introduction of an interprofessional oral health curriculum. J Physician Assist Educ 2015;26(1):43–6.

40. Wall T, Vujicic M. Emergency department use for dental conditions continues to increase. Health policy institute research brief. American Dental Association; 2015. Available at: http://www.ada.org/~/media/ADA/Science%20and%20Research/HPI/Files/HPIBrief_0415_2.ashx. Accessed May 14, 2017.

41. American Dental Association - Action For dental health. ER referral model summary. Available at: http://www.ada.org/~/media/ADA/Public%20Programs/Files/ER_Referral_Models_Summary_Flyer.pdf?la=en. Accessed May 14, 2017.

42. Pierce KM, Rozier RG, Vann WF Jr. Accuracy of pediatric primary care providers' screening and referral for early childhood caries. Pediatrics 2002;109:E82–92.

43. Achembong LN, Kranz AM, Rozier RG. Office-based preventive dental program and statewide trends in dental caries. Pediatrics 2014;133:e827–34.

44. Ramos-Gomez FJ, Crystal YO, Ng MW, et al. Pediatric dental care: prevention and management protocols based on caries risk assessment. J Calif Dent Assoc 2010;38(10):746–61.

45. Raths D. Teledentistry making a difference in rural New York. Healthcare informatics. 2015. Available at: http://www.healthcare-informatics.com/blogs/david-raths/teledentistry-making-difference-rural-new-york. Accessed May 14, 2017.

46. Project ECHO. http://echo.unm.edu/. Accessed May 14, 2017.

47. Arizona Alliance for Community Health Centers. A guide to promoting oral health in community health centers and achieving medical-dental integration. Available at: http://www.aachc.org/wp-content/uploads/2014/04/AACHC Oral-Health-Toolkit_3rd-Edition.pdf. Accessed May 14, 2017.

48. Doherty M. Safety net solutions – DentaQuest Institute. When two become one: models of the collaboration and integration of primary care and oral health. April 2012. National Oral Health Conference. Available at: http://www.nationaloralhealthconference.com/docs/presentations/2012/05-02/Mark%20Doherty.pdf. Accessed May 14, 2017.

49. Speare Memorial Hospital 2013 Annual Report, Ruth Doerric, page 8. Available at: http://www.spearehospital.com/wp-content/uploads/2013/10/SM-144-AR-2013-AR-web.pdf. Accessed May 14, 2017.

50. Harvard School of Dental Medicine and Northeastern University School of Nursing collaborate on a $1.2 Million HRSA-funded program that aims to bring primary care services into a dental care practice. Harvard School of Dental Medicine website. Available at: http://hsdm.harvard.edu/news/harvard-school-dental-medicine-and-northeastern-university-school-nursing-collaborate-12. Accessed May 14, 2017.

51. Greenberg BL, Glick M, Frantsve-Hawley J, et al. Dentists' attitudes toward chairside screening for medical conditions. J Am Dent Assoc 2010;141(1):52–62.
52. Greenberg BL, Thomas PA, Glick M, et al. Physicians' attitudes toward medical screening in a dental setting. J Public Health Dent 2015;75(3):225–33.
53. Greenberg BL, Kantor ML, Jiang SS, et al. Patients' attitudes toward screening for medical conditions in a dental setting. J Public Health Dent 2012;72(1):28–35.
54. American Board of Pediatrics, content outline, general pediatrics, certification examination. Page 56-57 section XXIII ears, nose and throat disorders E. 3. Mouth and oro-pharynx. Available at: https://www.abp.org/sites/abp/files/pdf/blueprint_gp_2016.pdf. Accessed May 14, 2017.
55. Integrating medical-dental care coordination for diabetic patients: a pilot effort. AACSP annual symposium 2014. Available at: http://aacdp.com/docs/2014Symposium/Acharya.pdf. Accessed May 14, 2017.
56. Leavett Partners. Dental care in accountable care organizations: insights from 5 case studies. Available at: http://www.ada.org/~/media/ADA/Science%20and%20Research/HPI/Files/HPIBrief_0615_1.ashx. Accessed May 14, 2017.
57. Massachusetts Medical Society Committee on Oral Health. Available at: http://www.massmed.org/Governance-and-Leadership/Committees,-Task-Forces-and-Sections/Committee-on-Oral-Health/#.VqTd8iorLIUS. Accessed May 14, 2017.
58. American Academy of Family Physicians Oral Health Member Interest Group. Available at: http://www.aafp.org/about/member-interest-groups/mig/oral-health.html. Accessed May 14, 2017.
59. Kelley BF, Sicilia JM, Forman S, et al. Advanced procedural training in family medicine: a group consensus statement. Fam Med 2009;41(6):398–404. Available at: https://www.stfm.org/fmhub/fm2009/June/Barbara398.pdf. Accessed May 14, 2017.
60. Zezima K. Short of dentists, Maine adds teeth to doctors' training. New York Times 2009. Available at: http://www.nytimes.com/2009/03/03/us/03dentist.html?_r=0. Accessed May 14, 2017.
61. American Academy of Pediatrics. Education in Quality Improvement for Pediatric Practice (EQIPP). Oral health and primary care. Available at: http://eqipp.aap.org/. Accessed May 14, 2017.

Fluorides and Other Preventive Strategies for Tooth Decay

Jeremy A. Horst, DDS, PhD[a], Jason M. Tanzer, DMD, PhD, DHC[b], Peter M. Milgrom, DDS[c],*

KEYWORDS

- Fluorides • Topical • Public health dentistry • Dental caries • Silver diamine fluoride
- Pit and fissure sealants

KEY POINTS

- Scarce public health resources should be directed toward intensive prevention of dental caries in toddlers and preschool-aged children.
- Expansion of school programs to include more strategies to atraumatically arrest lesions would increase program effectiveness.
- The risk and the need for primary prevention are not static but change across the life course.
- Public water and salt fluoridation, and taxes on sugar consumption are cost-effective approaches to decrease risk and increase resistance. Fluoride toothpaste should be distributed widely.
- Fluoride is not sufficient to control dental caries in high-risk patients. Topical antimicrobial therapies and dietary modifications should be instituted.

This article focuses on strategies to reduce the burden of dental caries across the population, using fluorides and some other dental caries preventive agents. It is imperative to be purposeful about the goals of using the various interventions, and particularly that agents should be targeted by patterns of disease susceptibility, which are

Disclosure Statement: J.A. Horst declares no conflict of interest. P.M. Milgrom is a director of Advantage Silver Dental Arrest, LLC, and served as a consultant to Cadbury Ltd and Kraft Foods Inc. J.M. Tanzer has served as a grant reviewer for the Sugar Association and the National Dairy Council and as a consultant for BASF and Advantage Silver Arrest, LLC.

a Department of Biochemistry and Biophysics, University of California San Francisco, 1700 4th Street, QB3 Room 404, San Francisco, CA 94158, USA; b Section on Oral Medicine, Department of Oral and Maxillofacial Diagnostic Sciences, University of Connecticut Health, University of Connecticut, 263 Farmington Avenue, Farmington, CT 06030, USA; c Department of Oral Health Sciences, University of Washington, Box 357475, Seattle, WA 98195-7475, USA
* Corresponding author.
E-mail address: dfrc@uw.edu

Dent Clin N Am 62 (2018) 207–234
https://doi.org/10.1016/j.cden.2017.11.003
0011-8532/18/© 2017 Elsevier Inc. All rights reserved.

associated with age. Dental caries in its various forms—early childhood caries (ECC), severe ECC, primary dental caries of the deciduous and permanent dentition, recurrent caries, and root surface caries—are diseases in which the products of sugar metabolism by certain bacteria that populate the tooth surface induce the development and progression of lesions.

These lesions (so-called cavities) are the clinical expression of disease, in which dental plaque bacteria metabolize sugar into polymeric substances that stabilize their adherence to the tooth and into acids that demineralize the hard tissues of the tooth. The term caries lesion includes the spectrum of lost tooth structure ranging from "white spot" enamel demineralizations, through large cavitations that extend into dentin. The bacterial species involved in the disease process are substantially known, but vary among depths and sites of caries lesions. There is little evidence that any interventions currently in use by dentists reduce the incidence of dental caries as a disease. The most effective interventions now known decrease the incidence of new lesions and curtail lesion growth, and these will be a major subject of this article. Dentists, it should be noted, currently spend most of their time dealing with previously treated caries lesions, referred to as recurrent or secondary caries lesions. Population-focused prevention efforts seek to alter the dental plaque biofilm, by reducing dietary sugar exposure, and improving the resilience of the teeth.

In general, primary prevention attempts to address etiology, and secondary prevention aims to stop progress of disease. Confusion arises from failure to distinguish the difference between tooth-level (lesion) versus individual- and population-level (disease) prevention. We do not have adequate, facile means to detect caries activity before lesions have occurred; the apparent breakdown of tooth structures is a result of a disease process that started earlier. The presence of visible lesions is the best available diagnostic for disease and predictor of future disease, so this is what we use. Meanwhile, cure of caries is just as elusive as for most cancers or coronary heart disease; what we presently do is count the years since the last sign of disease, such as the appearance of a new lesion or growth of an existing lesion. Thus, once a person has had any caries lesions it is unclear whether intervention could target primary prevention of disease. The aim in this case is to reduce the impact of the disease, that is, secondary prevention.

This paper focuses primarily on interventions that enhance resistance to disease progress. Enhancing resistance is achieved through the use of various fluorides, sugar substitutes, and mechanical barriers such as pit-and-fissure sealants. Relatively new to the discussion of primary and secondary prevention is the use of antimicrobials. Other key aspects of caries control are behavioral interventions (eg, motivational interviewing) with patients and their caretakers (parents, guardians, grandparents, etc) to promote use of disease transmission-reducing and resistance-enhancing agents. Behavioral intervention is necessary, because the interventions do have to be used to work.

A key means of risk reduction for primary prevention of dental caries on the population level is through a decrease of frequency and duration of exposure to dietary sugar. Such public health efforts—through present and potential government policies and industry food guidelines to improve overall nutrition—need to be part of dental public health practice. The enormous increases in sugars consumption over the past 40 years, and concomitant increase of human metabolic diseases (diabetes, obesity, heart disease, and stroke) demonstrate that people and families generally are not able to control sugar intake on their own, and thus system-wide public health changes are needed. However, efforts of the sugar industry during the 1960s and 1970s resulted in a shift away from research and progress in this field[1]; however, more recently, successful reductions in sugar consumption have been achieved by raising taxes, as in Mexico.[2]

Secondary prevention of caries requires early diagnosis and prompt treatment to reduce lesions' complications (pain, abscess, systemic infection, etc) and the occurrence of new lesions. Secondary prevention encompasses the concept of caries lesion arrest, because lesions that continue to grow can cause pain, tooth loss, and may serve as a reservoir of cariogenic bacteria that can initiate new lesions; antimicrobials are logical interventions. Lesions that grow also lead to escalating personal and public expense to replace parts of the dentition or, eventually, all of the dentition. The cascade of disfigurement of the dentition can impact social acceptance, growth patterns, and quality of life.[3] School-based screenings have been an important and widespread approach to early detection in secondary prevention, but have generally not led to either early diagnosis or prompt treatment, primarily because referrals are largely ineffective.[4] All school programs would be more effective if they used additional secondary prevention strategies to nonsurgically arrest lesions (as discussed elsewhere in this article).

TIMING OF PREVENTION EFFORTS
Children

The timing for the primary prevention of ECC (caries lesions in the primary dentition), to prevent the transmission of cariogenic bacteria to children, should be focused on mitigation and prevention of colonization of the dental biofilm (plaque) by cariogenic bacteria, especially *Streptococcus mutans*, which occurs within a couple years after tooth eruption. The child's mother or other caregivers, through transmission of salivary bacteria, is the usual source of *S mutans* that colonize young children.[5,6] When new mothers have low salivary *S mutans* levels, their babies' colonization by these bacteria is greatly delayed, as is the age and severity of caries lesions in those children; whereas, when mothers have high salivary *S mutans* levels, most of their babies are colonized younger and lesions occur within a couple of years thereafter.[5]

There is also good evidence that habitual maternal use of xylitol chewing gum during the first years of life of the infant protects the child from *S mutans* colonization, and the children get 71% to 78% fewer caries lesions (**Table 1**).[6–8] Thus, the first intervention should start with the caregivers, before the child has teeth.

Typically, cavities begin to appear early in the third year of life. In communities with very high disease burden, cavities appear within the first year after tooth eruption.

Table 1
Prevention of caries lesions in children by treating mothers with xylitol gum

First Author, Publication Year	Pubmed ID	Mother–Child Dyads	Age at Start (mo)	Xylitol Frequency	Duration of Intervention	Evaluation Time	Control	Prevented Fraction (%)
Isokangas et al,[9] 2000	11145360	195	3	4/d	21 mo	5 years old	NaF 2/y	71
Alamoudi et al,[7] 2014	24888659	60	10–36	3/d	3 mo	2 y later	NaF 2/y	78
Thorild et al,[6] 2006	17164069	173	6	3/d	1 y	4 years old	NaF/xylitol/ sorbitol	71

Abbreviation: NaF, sodium fluoride.

Primary prevention aimed at increasing tooth resistance must begin before this, when children are unlikely to see a dentist. S mutans and other cariogenic bacteria are unable to stably colonize the mouth until the teeth erupt, although they have been detected in the mouths of predentate children.[9] Thus, intensive prevention efforts for children in high-risk communities should start with female care deliverers before the time when teeth of their children erupt and continue after the teeth have come into the mouth, generally late in the first year of life. Scarce resources for dental public health are being deployed during preschool (eg, Head Start, 3–5 years old), often with the mistaken notion that this is primary prevention; the disease has already manifested by this age.

With each newly exposed tooth surface that enters the mouth, the opportunity presents for colonization by cariogenic bacteria. In permanent teeth, lesions typically follow 2 to 4 years after eruption (**Fig. 1**).[10] Often the rationale for the justification of efforts focused on the prevention and treatment of caries in primary teeth is the overstated connection of caries in primary teeth to that in permanent teeth; the contribution is very small with relative risk ratios such as 2.6[11] and 1.4.[12] Thankfully, children are in school at this age and easier to reach through school-based delivery systems. Although intensive interventions to get high-risk children into dental clinics have raised annual dental clinic visits from, approximately 12% to 43%,[13] bringing dental care to

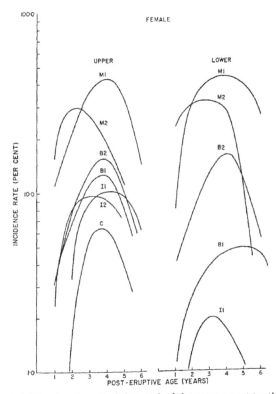

Fig. 1. Annual probability of caries attack (100 Q_x) of the permanent teeth, female children, Kingston, New York. Semilogarithmic scale. Probabilities are slightly lower in male children. B1, first bicuspid; B2, second bicuspid; C, canine; I1, central incisor; I2, lateral incisor; M1, first molar; M2, second molar. (*From* Carlos JP, Gittelsohn AM. Longitudinal studies of the natural history of caries—II. Arch Oral Biol 1965;10(5):745; with permission.)

schools is a more viable option for secondary prevention of decay of permanent teeth. Nonrestorative and minimally invasive options are logical treatments for primary teeth and early erupting permanent teeth. The grand opportunity afforded by exfoliation is to slow lesions in the primary dentition until the teeth shed, while preventing lesions in the permanent dentition. The importance of this goal cannot be overstated.

Adults

The majority of dental treatment in adults is the consequence of failure of fillings placed earlier in life; most fillings are replacements, owing to "recurrent caries" at the margins of or under old restorations. Dentists attribute the failures to the filling materials, but significant evidence to the contrary is now in the literature.[14,15] Excising lesions with a dental drill neither stops the initiation of new lesions, nor eliminates caries risk factors that led to the failure. Regardless, preventing recurrence is not primary prevention at either the disease or tooth level. In contrast, altering patient resistance to coronal and root caries is primary prevention of lesions when the effort is focused especially on those at greatest risk.

A major increase in the focus of public health efforts in adults should be on those who are transitioning into higher caries risk status, for example, when the quality and quantity saliva decreases (xerostomia) owing to polypharmacy, radiation exposure of the salivary glands, methamphetamine abuse, Sjögren's disease, and so on. In addition, root exposure after overbrushing and iatrogenic root surface damage attendant to mechanical instrumentation with the intent to control gingivitis and periodontal disease, and restoration of caries lesions that inadvertently damages the gingival attachment to the teeth and leads to root exposure, increase the number of at risk surfaces.

Efforts at the population level for adults are uncommon. Perhaps, to be effective, preventive interventions should be tied to other care encounters (periodontal care, primary medical care, and therapy for long term conditions such as substance abuse, heart disease, etc) so that the seminal risk-increasing events (drug abuse, chemotherapy, onset of systemic disease, multiple prescriptions) are addressed before damage is seen. Senior centers (>60 years) and subsidized public housing for elders (eg, HUD housing), assisted living, and skilled nursing facilities for older adults might be the focus of these efforts. The risk and the need for primary prevention are not static, but change across the life course.

PREVENTION AND ARREST: APPROACHES DURING EARLY CHILDHOOD

Caries does not occur without sugar. Rather, the evidence is overwhelming that the frequency of sugar consumption and the duration of sugar in the mouth are more powerful determinants of caries risk than is the quantity of its consumption.[16,17] Providing dietary guidance in dental public health programs at the earliest ages is imperative. Additionally, avoidance of sugar-enriched beverages such as juice drinks, sodas, and sports drinks at all ages is important, and the fallback strategy of rinsing with water after consumption of these artificial drinks are consumed may be useful, and should be studied further. Milk and baby formula should never be supplemented with sugar.

Patients with severe plaque owing to a complete lack of oral hygiene, but fed solely through gastric tubes or intravenous ports, do not get caries lesions. Likewise, patients with the genetic defects of intestinal sucrase deficiency or hereditary fructose intolerance (fructose is one-half of the sucrose molecule), who therefore avoid dietary sucrose do not develop appreciable caries lesions and have barely detectable *S mutans* in their mouths.[18,19] An increased frequency of simple sugar intake seems to have the greatest effect on the initiation of lesions. "Baby bottle tooth decay" resulting from cow's milk or artificial "formula" is an important example: restriction of milk bottle exposure to 3 to 6 meal times depending on weight and age reduces the incidence of caries dramatically, and exposure throughout the night is to be strongly discouraged.[20]

It takes time for cariogenic dental plaque to accumulate to the point when it can deliver enough acid onto the tooth surface to dissolve enamel. Cavities do not occur in constantly cleaned teeth. Frequently disturbing plaque by any means works to prevent caries lesions.[21] Caregivers need to be taught how to clean the teeth while maintaining reasonable comfort for all involved. It is helpful to build a sense of control in the child by breaking up each episode of brushing into small bits with structured time (counting), even during infancy. Teeth can be cleaned anywhere. Sinks and bathrooms are not needed and it is frequently easier to clean a young child's teeth on the floor or a sofa with the child's head on one's lap or between one's legs (**Fig. 2**).

Fluoride varnish decreases the amount of new caries lesions in school-aged children by 37%.[22] This effect was assumed to extrapolate to younger children. We ourselves had this hope, and documented the safety of fluoride varnish in infants.[23] A surge in fluoride varnish use starting with the eruption of the first tooth has come in the last decade, but positive results have not followed. **Table 2** details the outcomes of clinical trials on caries lesion prevention by fluoride varnish when starting the intervention before the third birthday. Disappointingly, 5 of the 6 studies using fluoride varnish alone show no prevention of new lesions.[24–30] The 3 studies that combine fluoride

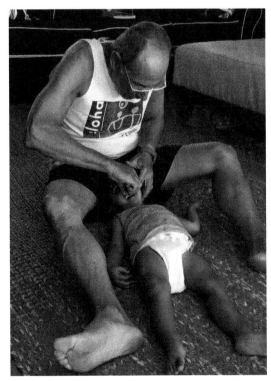

Fig. 2. One of the authors (PMM) brushing his grandson's teeth with fluoridated toothpaste.

Table 2
Prevention of caries lesions with fluoride varnish in children starting at 1 to 3 years of age

First Author, Publication Year	Pubmed ID	Children in Study	Age at Start (mo)	Frequency (Annual)	Duration (y)	Combined Intervention	Prevented Fraction (%)
Slade et al,[32] 2011	20707872	666	18–47	2	2	Guidance	31
Lawrence et al,[28] 2008	18422711	1275	6–71	2	2	None	25
Tickle et al,[31] 2016	27685609	1248	24–48	2	3	F toothpaste	25
Ramos-Gomez et al,[30] 2012	21999806	361	12–36	2	2	Maternal CHX	None
Jiang et al,[24] 2014	25448437	450	8–23	2	2	None	None
Agouropoulos et al,[25] 2014	25123352	424	24–71	2	2	None	None
Oliveira et al,[26] 2014	24481085	200	12–59	2	2	None	None
Memarpour et al,[27] 2015	25895964	140	12–36	3	1	None	None
Anderson et al,[29] 2016	26795957	3403	12	2	2	None	None

Nine recent clinical trials evaluated prevented fraction of caries lesions in toddlers, documenting an unfortunate lack of effect.
Abbreviations: CHX, chlorhexidine; F, fluoride.

varnish with other interventions also showed no effect, or only the expected effect of the other interventions.[31,32]

One interpretation of this surprising disparity in the effectiveness of caries prevention by fluoride varnish at different ages is that differing balances of pathogenic and protective factors may occur at different ages. Perhaps dietary sugars, hygiene, and the composition of the dental plaque play a greater role than the enhancement of remineralization potential by fluoride varnish. It may also be that diverse varnishes vary in their effectiveness; no clinical testing has been done on the preventive effect of most fluoride varnishes currently on the market.[33] The lack of effect observed in these recent trials deserves further study. For now, we recommend use of interventions that consistently show an effect.

Promising work has been done on the combination of antimicrobial agents with fluoride varnish. Two clinical studies in toddlers (12–35 month old) show an added benefit of painting povidone iodine onto the teeth immediately before the fluoride varnish, every 2 to 4 months for at least 10 months. As summarized in **Table 3**, a clinical trial resulted in 80% fewer children having any signs of caries after 1 year of bimonthly combined iodine-fluoride treatment, as compared with fluoride varnish only.[34] A cluster intervention showed that inclusion of povidone iodine resulted in 24% fewer children having any signs of disease after 10 months with approximately 2.5 treatments per child, and 31% fewer new lesions total.[35] The prevention of caries by antimicrobials is understudied in infants and toddlers.

Fluoride supplement tablets show 24% prevention of caries lesions in permanent teeth, but such an effect has not proven to be consistent for primary teeth, and the

Table 3
Prevention of dental caries by placement of povidone iodine before fluoride varnish in toddlers

First Author, Publication Year	Pubmed ID	Patients	Age at Start (mo)	Frequency (Annual)	Duration of Intervention	Follow-up	Control	Notes	Preventec Fraction (%)
Lopez et al,[34] 2002	12064491	72	12–19 mo	Every 2 mo	1 y	1 y	F Varnish Only	—	80
Amin et al,[133] 2004	15080351	25	2–7 y	Every 2 mo	6 mo	1 y	None	Post-GA, no F varnish	71
Simratvir et al,[134] 2010	20578661	30	μ = 4.2 y	Every 3 mo	1 y	1 y	Water	Post-GA, no F varnish	100
Tut & Milgrom,[100] 2010	20337902	614	5–6 y	Every 4 mo	10 mo	10 mo	F Varnish Only	—	46
Milgrom et al,[35] 2011	22126926	172	12–30 mo	Every 4 mo	10 mo	10 mo	F varnish only	—	24
Xu et al,[135] 2009	19417885	61	6–9 y	Every 1 wk	1 mo	1 y	Foam	Foam iodine, no F varnish	0
Zhan et al,[98] 2006	16913243	22	2–6 y	Once	Once	1 y	PBS, F gel	Post-GA, F gel	0

Abbreviations: F, fluoride; GA, general anesthesia; PES, phosphate-buffered saline; μ, mean.

effect is no greater than topical fluoride rinses, varnish, or toothpaste, which presumably pose less risk of fluorosis.[36] If this is to be done, it is wise—especially if the children drink well water—that parents determine the level of fluoride in that water.

COMMUNITY FLUORIDATION

After the discovery of the preventive effects of fluoride in water against dental caries, fluoride was added to water, milk, and salt. The scalability (amenability to general implementation) of this intervention arises from centralized production and existing government regulation of these vehicles. Water fluoridation is the most widely adopted, reaching more than 370 million people in 27 countries, with many studies demonstrating effectiveness and safety, with the sole exception of dental fluorosis as a possible side effect. The cost is roughly 20 to 50 cents per person per year in the United States.[37] A recent Cochrane metaanalysis included 107 studies with an estimated average of 35% prevented fraction of caries lesions in the primary dentition (dmft), 26% prevention of lesions in permanent teeth (DMFT), and 15% prevention of any new lesions (primary disease prevention). The authors caution, however, that 72 of the studies were conducted before the widespread use of fluoride toothpaste, and that benefit from the combination is uncertain. Nevertheless, prevention by fluoride toothpaste is independent of fluoridated water exposure, so one might expect a combined benefit. Twelve percent of recipients have esthetic concerns about dental fluorosis attributable to water fluoridation.[38]

Salt fluoridation reaches about 60 million people in Europe and more than 100 million in Latin America including Mexico. The cost is one-tenth of water fluoridation, making it by far the least expensive and probably the most efficient method of caries prevention. Although no modern clinical trials on the caries preventive effects of salt fluoridation are known to us, older cluster-randomized studies consistently show 50% prevention of new lesions.[39]

Milk fluoridation offers the highest precision of fluoride dose, because the variation in quantity of milk intake is lower among children than that for tap water or salt, and can be further metered by single serving boxes. The cost is US $1 to $2.50 per person per year, roughly 5 times that of water fluoridation. Accordingly, only about 1 million children receive fluoridated milk.[40] Despite many demonstration projects, a recent Cochrane review found only one placebo-controlled clinical trial of milk fluoridation, in which a 31% prevented fraction was observed in the primary dentition; the lesion increment in the permanent dentition of the control group was too low to make any conclusions.[41]

The reported target of these scalable fluoridation interventions generally was children. However, impact across the age spectrum can be achieved. In countries that predominantly consume processed food (such as the United States, Mexico, and Canada) and have a high prevalence of dental caries, physicians recommend limiting salt intake owing to exacerbation of hypertension associated with cardiovascular disease. Gestational hypertension bears the same concerns. Thus, although the cost effectiveness is provocative, the propriety of salt fluoridation for older adults or pregnant women should be approached with caution and further study. Most countries curtail milk consumption during later childhood. Community water fluoridation, therefore, seems to be the large, scalable intervention of choice to prevent caries during adulthood.

THE IMPORTANCE OF FLUORIDE TOOTHPASTE

The sale of fluoride toothpaste has been profoundly successful. In the United States, an average of 3 tubes of toothpaste are sold for every person annually. Across 70 clinical trials, 24% of caries lesions are prevented by using fluoride toothpaste compared with nonfluoride toothpaste, and this effect is not decreased by exposure to fluoridated water. Metaanalysis by concentration of fluoride shows a dose response that seems to reach maximum effect at 37% prevented lesions for the highest tested concentrations: 2400 to 2800 ppm F. Disease-level prevention (no new lesions) is seen in 12% of patients using over-the-counter (OTC) strength fluoride toothpastes, 1000 to 1500 ppm in primary or permanent teeth, compared with controls.[42] Significant heterogeneity in disease-level outcomes is seen. No placebo-controlled trials have been conducted in 30 years, although the free fluoride concentrations in these toothpastes have increased. One trial, conducted before the inception of adding fluoride into toothpaste, observed a 25% decrease in caries lesions with calcium phosphate toothpaste versus no toothpaste. Brushing without a dentifrice or with a dentifrice without fluoride has long been assumed to have an important effect on lesion prevention, but numerous trials have shown a lack of prevention of new lesions, even in supervised studies. Unquestionably, brushing per se inhibits gingivitis and that is a major reason dental providers stress its importance.

Children's toothpastes (850–1150 ppm fluoride) for those under 6 years of age (when mineralization of all tooth crowns except the second permanent molars has been completed), and pastes with as much as 5000 ppm F for older children or adults, are effective self-administered topical drugs for primary prevention of tooth decay. The efficacy of these self-applied fluorides has been particularly well-documented in trials in the young permanent dentition in a wide range of populations (as discussed elsewhere in this article). As mentioned, the prevalence of dental caries lesions decreases by 20% to 30% in populations using fluoridated toothpaste. Supervised tooth brushing in schools is effective. Rinsing is not encouraged generally after normal brushing, as exemplified by the Oral Health Foundation's "Spit don't rinse" slogan.

Free postal delivery of toothpaste along with advice from home visitors not only reduces decay at the 24% rate seen in trials with direct administration, but reduces need for dental extractions in lower socioeconomic groups.[43] Therefore, the distribution of toothpaste ultimately reduces pain, disfigurement, and further, more extensive and costly complications of caries, which are important goals. Although successfully implemented at other ages, toothpaste use has not been effective as a public health measure in preventing ECC. Although the American Dental Association recommends that appropriate amounts of fluoride toothpaste be used for high-risk children of all ages,[44] many health care workers continue to discourage early adoption of fluoridated toothpaste to reduce the risk of fluorosis. However, a retrospective study of an Australian population exposed to fluoride toothpaste early in life shows a relatively small increase in fluorosis, and at the same time demonstrates extensive protection against tooth decay. The highest metaanalysis estimate of increased risk of fluorosis by toothpaste is 2-fold.[45] Most fluorosis is of no clinical significance. Furthermore, fluorosis is not related to quality-of-life measures.[46] If fluorosis concerns persist, roughly one-third less fluorosis occurs when delaying use until after the first birthday.[44,45]

Parents need guidance from primary care providers about how to choose a fluoride-containing toothpaste. They are confused by the labeling and advertising. They also need instruction on how to brush a child's teeth. Often parents think they need to brush the teeth in the bathroom awkwardly trying to do this with the child sitting on the sink. They cannot see the teeth or keep the mouth open. Many parents and caregivers think that children can brush their own teeth, even when they are very young. They need to be taught that a parent should model good brushing, and also brush the child's teeth themselves until the surprisingly old age when children can effectively brush (circa 7 years). Some parents believe that the teeth may be damaged by brushing, or that 3-year-olds can brush properly: parents need accurate information.

FLUORIDE RINSES, FOAMS, VARNISH, AND HIGH FLUORIDE TOOTHPASTES AND GELS

Clearly, fluoride can prevent caries lesions in school-aged children and older adults in any of the available delivery systems—26% by lesion, and 12% by disease.[47] Industry and academic efforts to optimize benefits have focused on minimizing application frequency and protocol duration, while maximizing the prevented fraction of caries lesions. Massive development efforts have gone into the various delivery approaches: rinses, varnishes, foams, gels, and so on. Varnish seems to be the endpoint of single-agent fluoride-only materials, because the protocol demands only seconds, varnish can be favorably flavored, and twice per year application seems to maximize the effect. Still, the greater use of foams may be owing to their more favorable textures. Although daily fluoride exposure may contribute to the control of dental plaque bacteria, it must be remembered that professionally applied fluorides operate mostly by increasing the remineralization of the enamel surface. It is not surprising that these single agent therapies top out at approximately 37% prevention. In view of the small differences in effects between topical fluorides, it is not surprising that adoption is so low, even 20 years after the introduction of fluoride varnish to the United States. According to industry experts, it is estimated that only one-half of dental offices use fluoride varnish (Kevin Thomas of Elevate Oral Care, personal communication, 2016).

Fluoride rinses result in 27% fewer lesions, or 23% fewer permanent teeth with lesions.[48] Rinsing with fluoride instead of brushing with it achieves similar outcomes.[49] Rinsing with fluoride may be particularly useful for prevention in teenagers or others who are old enough to rinse but have trouble with motivation or dexterity to brush, because rinsing is simpler. Only 1 study of fluoride varnish explicitly in addition to fluoride toothpaste has been done, although most studies of varnish to prevent lesions in children occurred in the background of fluoride toothpaste; their effects were equivalent. No significant differences are seen among rinses, gels, varnishes, and toothpastes in the few available studies,[49] although these studies seem to be too small to have been able to detect a difference if one had existed. Not accounting for the recent studies in 1- to 3-year-old children (summarized in **Table 2**), the prevented fraction of lesions estimated for each topical fluoride is as follows: daily OTC toothpaste 24%, daily prescription (5000 ppm) toothpaste 37%, daily rinse 26%, semiannual gel 21%, and semiannual varnish 37%.[42,47]

Considering the cost effectiveness and additive benefit, the best approach to using fluoride for primary prevention as the risk increases seems to be normal strength fluoride toothpaste until the completion of permanent tooth crown formation (circa 8 years), then 5000 ppm fluoride toothpaste, each together with fluoride varnish 2 times per year.

Stannous fluoride in toothpaste has been understudied, perhaps because of concerns about tooth surface staining and taste. The color change of the dentition's surface is probably owing to oxidized porphyrins from dead bacteria and oxidized tin. There is some evidence of effectiveness, but none of the studies are modern, placebo-controlled, randomized, clinical trials. Blinding of examiners and participants is problematic. Meanwhile, the potential activity of the tin ion against dental caries in available OTC products should be evaluated further.

SILVER DIAMINE FLUORIDE AS A TREATMENT AND PREVENTIVE FOR CARIES

Silver diamine fluoride is a topical treatment for caries lesions and a primary preventive for newly exposed, high-risk surfaces, such as first molar fissures or roots.[50] Its mechanism(s) of action is under investigation. However, silver diamine fluoride has double the concentration of fluoride (approximately 5%) as that in varnish, is 25% weight/volume silver ions, and has 8% ammonia, in water.[51] It is currently presumed that the high fluoride content allows for more effective diffusion into enamel and dentin, that the silver kills bacteria upon contact, and differentially stays in demineralized or hypomineralized tooth structures, both hardening the structures and reactivating upon exposure to bacterial metabolic byproducts, thereby preventing their reinvasion, and that the ammonia stabilizes the solution and serves as an antiseptic to add to microbial kill on contact.[52–54] This hypothesized triple mechanism seems well-suited for caries because this material treats the disease etiology.

Clearance by the US Food and Drug Administration (FDA) in 2014 and availability of the product in 2015 have catalyzed adoption. No dental product has had such rapid adoption. We estimate that 16 to 20% of US dentists now have a supply. Canada approved the same product in early 2017 and 10% have a supply. The FDA recently designated silver diamine fluoride with Breakthrough Therapy Status, which is a commitment to a drug application for a serious disease for which there is no medical treatment and great public health need.

Nine clinical trials document caries arrest by treatment of cavitated dentin lesions with silver diamine fluoride in children and older adults. Twice per year application apparently maximizes the arrest effect that increases to 90% after 2 years of treatment.[55,56] Maintenance of arrest seems to depend on at least annual reapplication.[57,58] Furthermore, after 2.5 to 3.0 years, 70% fewer lesions are observed on the untreated surfaces of patients whose lesions were treated with silver diamine fluoride.[55,59] This observation of fewer new lesions from treating only existing lesions seems to surpass that for operative treatment, which is approximately 38% after 2 years.[15] The prevention of new lesions is also documented, where application to high-risk surfaces once per year is equivalent to or more effective than fluoride varnish 4 times per year in children or older adults.[60,61]

The only known side effect of silver diamine fluoride is the staining of lesions. The silver tarnishes to black. This color change is an index of the effectiveness of the treatment, where the entire lesion turning black indicates success: all lesions that are completely black are apparently arrested. Some lesions that are arrested do not turn entirely black, but this is fairly obvious from the shiny dentin; all demineralized (carious) or hypomineralized dentin or enamel will stain black. Parents and caregivers generally do not object to the stains in primary teeth when the treatment is explained and the alternative is operative treatment.[62] The carious dentin is hardened by the treatment to twice normal dentin hardness.[63]

Application is simple (dry and apply), such that any dental or medical provider can provide the treatment. Nurses and hygienists who can provide care at remote sites such as schools or nursing homes should be encouraged to adopt silver diamine fluoride to manage dental caries lesions. Monitoring is simple. The cost of the material is commensurate with fluoride varnish.

SEALANTS FOR PRIMARY PREVENTION

Sealants form mechanical barriers that isolate the pits, grooves, and defects in the biting (occlusal) surfaces of the teeth from the dental plaque and dietary constituents. They also can fill defects in smooth surfaces. Sealants were developed in part because water fluoridation was not as effective a decay preventive on occlusal pit and fissure surfaces as on the smooth surfaces of the teeth (buccal, lingual, and proximal), and also to treat early lesions.[64]

Sealants continue to be used in public health even as evidence—both histologic and clinical—has mounted that topical fluorides are effective and less expensive. The placement of plastic resin sealants is a time-intensive and technique-sensitive proced-ure requiring skilled personnel and significant patient tolerance, for example, compared with application of topical fluorides. Effective resin sealant application in children requires 4 hands. Studies have shown no statistically significant difference in the preventive effects of resin sealants versus fluoride varnish.[65,66] Sealants in pub-lic health, placed on the basis of poverty status alone, are expensive, and may be an inefficient use of scarce resources. Nonetheless, a direct cost-effectiveness compar-ison is important, for example, to account for the consolidation of efforts into fewer visits by sealants than for topical fluorides. A recent study comparing the 2 treatments again showed no significant differences in the prevention of pit and fissure lesions by 6 monthly applications of fluoride varnish or sealants in first permanent molars, but a careful analysis showed cost savings of US \$88.53 (£68.13) per patient using the var-nish.[67] Also, resin sealants do not alter the risk for caries lesions on untreated sur-faces, whereas fluoride varnish is easily applied to other surfaces.

Although public health outreach efforts to deliver sealants for first permanent molars are successful, almost no similar efforts have been made to place sealants in second permanent molars. This lack of coverage of older children and adolescents is important because caries lesions that develop during adolescence often go untreated and can result in expensive visits to the emergency department of hospitals a decade later.[68]

Resin sealants are considered the standard of care for prevention of lesions on the treated surfaces, or as treatment for noncavitated lesions.[69] They should only be placed in children or adolescents who have clearly documented past caries experi-ence or large amounts of plaque on their teeth. The presence of fillings is not always a good indicator of past caries lesion experience because the diagnosis of caries le-sions among dentists is highly variable. The best indicator of dental caries is frank cavitation. Also, sealants may be indicated if a child has a medical condition that directly or indirectly impacts salivary flow, or where medications contain sugar, as in syrups. Although the focus is on first and second permanent molars, defects or deep fissures in primary molars in caries-active children merit the use of sealants.

Significant evidence suggests that the replacement of resin sealants by high viscos-ity glass ionomer cements should be considered. Glass ionomer cement sealants release fluoride and metal ions into the parts of the tooth most susceptible to caries, and do not require a dry field to be created in the moist environment of the mouth. When the bulk of the cement is lost, some material remains in the deepest parts of the grooves to provide mechanical protection. When lesions are used as an endpoint (instead of retention), resin and glass ionomer cement sealants show equivalence in metaanalyses at 2, 3, 4, and 5 years after placement.[70] There is a markedly greater ease of application: the tooth is brushed, then the material is mixed and pushed into the pits and grooves of all teeth. This increases the speed and therefore presum-ably the cost effectiveness. There is also evidence of superior prevention on untreated surfaces by glass ionomer cements. For example, a study of 2557 children in Italy demonstrated 35% prevention of caries lesions on the distal of the second primary molars when using glass ionomer cement compared with resin.[71] Because resin seal-ants will not be successful unless placed in a very dry field, glass ionomer cement sealants may offer a better alternative generally, and particularly if the molar tooth is erupting, the child is unable to cooperate, or if the operator is working alone. Patient preference and cost effectiveness should be studied further.

Resin sealants, when placed well, have a relatively high retention rate. However, the goal is not to retain a material; it is to prevent caries lesions. There is misunderstanding that the Oral Health 2020 goals state that sealants should be retained in certain percent-ages of children; the actual goals state that certain percentages of children should have their teeth sealed. The monitoring of sealant retention is a surrogate measure specific to resin sealants. The effectiveness of glass ionomer cement sealants does not rely on retention. Meanwhile, there is no innate therapeutic value to resin, such that leaking resin margins create a microenvironment that promotes tooth decay. Public health sealant programs have mistakenly been set up to monitor the surrogate marker of sealant presence rather than actual lesions as the response variable. These systems need to adapt to new data, and implement interventions that lead to the best clinical outcomes.

XYLITOL AND OTHER POLYOLS

Sugar substitutes have long been sought and some studied extensively: xylitol, a 5-carbon sugar alcohol has proved to have unexpected antibacterial effects specific for S mutans by compromising its metabolism and colonization.[72] Studies began with a remarkable series of mostly human clinical trials. In the Turku Sugar Studies, Scheinin and Mäkinen[73] substituted the nonfermentable polyol xylitol for virtually the entire sugar content of the dietary components of dental students and faculty at a dental school in Finland during a 3-year period. This substitution resulted in a remarkable caries incidence reduction, by comparison with similarly fructose-substituted and conventional sucrose-containing foods. Essentially, no new lesions were seen in the xylitol group, whereas 7.2 were gained in the sucrose group.[74] It is, however, impractical for humans to make such complete dietary substitutions owing to gastrointestinal intolerance to more than 50 g/d of xylitol, being a characteristic of all dietary additives or substitutes poorly absorbed from the gut.

Subsequently, controlled studies demonstrated that several exposures daily to high content xylitol-containing chewing gums or other confections with a high content of xylitol, thus greatly reducing the ingested load of xylitol (the remainder of the diet remaining essentially unaltered), also significantly inhibited caries prevalence and incidence. Notably, the greatest reduction of lesions occurred on the smooth surfaces of the teeth; the fissures and pits were least affected. The most remarkable of these longitudinal studies was carried out for 40 months with 10-year-olds in Belize, a society with a high sucrose consumption and high caries prevalence. Several studies have shown the biological bases of this effect to be essentially specific to the S mutans among the oral flora.[72] Some have argued that this anticaries effect of high-content xylitol gums is merely a reflection of sweet taste and gum chewing that increase salivary flow and salivary buffers, with the resultant clearance of food from the mouth and neutralization of acids in the plaque.[75] Nonetheless, the well-controlled Belize study that included gums of high content sorbitol alone and in combination with xylitol demonstrated a xylitol dose–response efficacy, and discounts this simple salivary flow and buffering explanation.[76] Additionally, large population studies of fluoride-containing toothpastes containing either 10% sorbitol or 10% xylitol also show an augmentation of decay-preventive effects of the fluoride when containing 10% xylitol.[77,78] A recent, smaller study did not show any benefit.[79] Mainstream toothpaste manufacturers in the United States do not presently make their pastes with xylitol. A recent study of xylitol lozenges in adults with low caries lesion backgrounds showed no effect on coronal lesions, but a reduction in root lesions.[80]

Other nonfermentable or slowly fermented (by dental plaque bacteria) sugar substitutes have been studied beside xylitol. Of long interest have been sorbitol and mannitol (6-carbon sugar alcohols, widely used in sugar-free confections in the United States) and inducibly transported and catabolized in part to ethanol[81]; they are associated with modest caries reduction consistent with partial substitution of sugar confections in the diet.[82] Erythritol (a 4-carbon sugar alcohol analog of xylitol), when added in high concentration to a glucose-containing culture medium, slows the growth of mutans streptococci, as does xylitol,[83] but unlike xylitol, it is not associated with a reduction of total streptococci in interdental plaque.[84] A 2-year cluster randomized trial in children at low risk for lesion development (average 1.5 new lesions after 2 years), drinking fluoridated water, observed no difference between lesion scores for lozenges that contained either xylitol–maltitol (4.7 g/d, 4.6 g/d total, respectively) or erythritol–maltitol (4.5 g/d, 4.2 g/d total) versus participants not given lozenges.[85] Maltosyl–erythritol, a triose alcohol, has been reported to inhibit extracellular glucan synthesis from sucrose by *Streptococcus sobrinus*, one of the mutans streptococci prevalent on human teeth, but we know of no clinical studies with it.[86] The other clinical trial of erythritol (7.5 g/d total) confections known to us showed prevention of caries lesions in children with respect to sorbitol or xylitol candies, although comparisons were performed on total lesions in each group rather than the standard change in DMFS, which deflates variance metrics and is, therefore, questionable.[87]

Also notable as a sugar substitute is isomaltitol (Palatinit, Isomalt) which is now prominent in sugar free confections in the United States and many other countries. It is a 1:1 mixture of 2 synthetic disaccharide alcohols, namely, glucosyl–sorbitol and glucosyl–mannitol. It is slowly fermentable,[88] claimed not to lower the pH in human dental plaque unlike sugars, and is reportedly noncariogenic in rats.[89] However, an extensive literature search reveals no clinical studies to date that indicate it either reduces *S mutans* colonization levels or reduces tooth decay incidence in humans.

Perhaps the most surprising and important public health data from studies of xylitol gum chewing come from the study of mothers who chewed xylitol gum daily postpartum, and whose initially 3-month-old infants experienced delayed colonization by mutans streptococci, and dramatically lower levels of carious lesions at 5 and 7 years of age, even though the mothers were instructed to stop chewing xylitol gum when their children were 15 month of age.[8] Confirmation of this pattern is seen in 2 other studies (see **Table 1**). These data are illustrative of primary prevention of caries by prevention of mother–child transmission of the prime pathogen of caries. Thus, it can reasonably be concluded that xylitol is of interest in the realms of primary and secondary prevention of tooth decay.

ANTIBIOTIC AND ANTISEPTIC AGENTS
Antibiotics and Immunization

Although chronic antibiotic use, as formerly common when rheumatic fever was prevalent in the United States, was noted to sharply decrease caries prevalence among penicillin users,[90] it is universally deemed inappropriate to use antibiotics to inhibit caries because of allergic sensitization of the host and because of the risk of spread of antibiotic resistance among bacteria. Considerable progress has been made in efforts to develop immunization against the mutans streptococci, a group-specific or species-specific approach to caries control, leaving the rest of the oral flora relatively unaffected. To date, almost all work has been done in nonhuman experimental animals and in vitro. A proposal for human trials of vaccine in the United Kingdom has been turned down by its FDA-analogous agency with its feeling that all vaccines carry some, albeit generally rare, risk of significant adverse effects on the host, such as Guillain-Barré syndrome, and that there already exist good nonimmunologic means to inhibit caries, including sugar restriction, fluorides, sealants, and so on. One must view the prospect of immunization against caries as distant.

Nonetheless, at least 1 patent for an immunologic has been sold to a drug company recently.

ANTISEPTIC AGENTS
Chlorhexidine and Combinations with Chlorhexidine

Several nonspecific, albeit potent, antiseptic agents have been of interest in the secondary prevention of caries affecting crown (enamel) and root (dentin) surfaces. The most studied has been chlorhexidine, which kills most bacteria rapidly by disruption of their cell walls. This antiseptic is available in different forms and concentrations in various countries. It is importantly benign to the host's mucous membranes and skin. An 0.20% mouth rinse was of initial interest in Scandinavia for its inhibition of supragingival dental plaque and associated gingivitis, for which it was effective even in the absence of tooth brushing and flossing. A nonrandomized study of caries inhibition using 1% chlorhexidine gel resulted in 56% fewer lesions after 3 years.[91] These studies, among others, led to attempts by a US company to introduce an OTC chlorhexidine mouth rinse, but the concentration of chlorhexidine that cleared the FDA was reduced to 0.12% and the product was required to be marketed by prescription only.

It was known by this time that chlorhexidine rinsing would reduce short-term salivary mutans streptococcal titers by 1000-fold, but that those titers rebound to baseline in about 3 months. This provided part of the rationale for a study of whether operative dentistry to surgically remove recurrent carious lesions after prolonged rinsing with 0.12% chlorhexidine could provide better outcomes if patients were to then chew either xylitol gum, sorbitol gum, or no gum for a period of 3 months. It was observed that xylitol gum greatly delayed the rebound of mutans streptococci in saliva, whereas sorbitol gum chewing had no effect; typical rebound occurred, as it did in the no gum control group.[92] This dramatized the prospective utility of xylitol gum for secondary caries prevention, and argued against the idea that its effects were attributable simply to saliva flow stimulation, as discussed elsewhere in this article.

Attempts have been made to deliver chlorhexidine in gels and varnishes to the teeth, with inconsistent demonstrations of efficacy. Fourteen clinical trials on the prevention of caries with chlorhexidine products have shown markedly different results. Although 3 trials using 1% chlorhexidine plus 1% thymol, or 10% chlorhexidine show an effect to prevent root caries, no effects were seen in metaanalysis of the other 5 clinical trials in older adults,[93] and the 8 in children.[94] Patients in the 3 trials showing an effect did not have access to routine prophylactic dental cleanings. The lack of effect seen for 40% chlorhexidine varnish was particularly concerning because a dose–response effect is expected for effective interventions. However, little or no evidence was reported that the chlorhexidine was released from the diverse matrices in these studies. The chlorhexidine may have been bound in the varnishes and never released; bioavailability needs to be tested before clinical trials. A large, carefully executed multicenter trial in the United States, in which chlorhexidine release from varnish was verified, demonstrated a lack of caries prevention for 10% chlorhexidine varnish in adults.[95]

In contrast, several chlorhexidine-containing vehicles have been shown in randomized trials to have an effect on caries lesions.[96] In a notable study, 1% chlorhexidine gel was applied to the teeth of teenagers using applicator trays for 1 min/d for 14 days, whenever their paraffin-stimulated salivary S mutans levels were greater than 2.5×10^5 cfu/mL, at baseline, and every 4 months thereafter. The strategy effected a short-term 2 to 3 log reduction of salivary titers, with long-term 1-log reductions only in those starting with titers of greater than 10^6 cfu/mL. Pit and fissure sealants were also placed at baseline in the intervention arm. All participants rinsed with 0.2% NaF every 2 weeks during the 3 school years of the study. There were 56% fewer lesions seen across all intervention group patients, and 81% fewer among participants with greater than 10^6 cfu/mL S mutans at the start of the study. Thus, treating the risk factor of cariogenic bacteria salivary titers with an antimicrobial illustrated efficacy.[91] Additionally, 2 placebo-controlled trials showed significant prevention of interproximal caries lesions by flossing 1% chlorhexidine gel between the teeth. One study of 12-year-olds applied the chlorhexidine by floss 4 times per year for 3 years, resulting in 42% fewer new lesions and 68% fewer new fillings in the interproximal surfaces, compared with placebo quinine-flavored floss and a no flossing control. The placebo floss group scores were not substantially different from the no flossing scores. No differences in S mutans salivary titers were noted.[91] An analogous study in 4-year-olds showed 43% fewer new lesions and 58% fewer new fillings in the interproximal surfaces.[97]

Iodine

Iodine-based disinfectants kill S mutans, albeit not selectively. They have long been accepted as skin and mucosal disinfectants, and seem to be extremely safe. Three clinical trials describe 1-time use in children in operative dental treatment under general anesthesia. This additional intervention lowers S mutans titers for approximately 6 months, but does not have an effect on clinical outcomes, as predicted by rebound of mutans levels.[98,99] However, repeated use of povidone iodine before fluoride varnish decreases the incidence of caries lesions (see **Table 3**). This is one of the only interventions that has been shown to work in toddlers that also works in school-aged children.[100]

Arginine

Safety and buffering of dental plaque owing to putative ionization of ammonium has led to interest in arginine somewhat recently. Various clinical trials ranging in size from 200 to 6000 participants on the use of toothpaste with 1.5% arginine, calcium carbonate, and fluoride all find nearly the same 20% reduction in caries lesions after 2 years compared with fluoride toothpaste.[101–103] Similar studies on the reversal or arrest of root caries lesions show some effect.[104,105] The effect is purported to be a metabolic shift away from acid production, and a change in the microbial profile toward health.[106] However, arginine has a strongly cationic guanidino functional group like the 2 guanidino groups of chlorhexidine, and thus may actually function as an antiseptic. Eight percent arginine-containing toothpastes are marketed by Colgate specifically to reduce dentin hypersensitivity in the United States, and toothpastes containing 1.5% arginine, calcium carbonate, and fluoride are available elsewhere. The manufacturer indicates that the product is safe for children.

OTHER AGENTS

Fluoride, silver, xylitol, chlorhexidine with thymol, povidone iodine, and arginine all seem to be effective agents and, to some degree, function in an antibacterial manner. Also, a myriad of papers describe kill of S mutans with extracts from natural products, such as high-molecular-weight cranberry extracts and numerous botanicals from Asia. Vitamin D also deserves more attention: 24 clinical studies on caries lesion prevention by vitamin D supplementation were conducted between the 2 World Wars, of which metaanalysis estimates 53% prevention.[107] The belief at the time of these studies was that vitamin D enhanced the quality of saliva. Work in Canada demonstrated a relationship between both maternal and children's blood vitamin D levels and caries experience.[108,109] This, however, was not observed in the US nationwide National Health and Nutrition Examination Survey data.[110] Although vitamin D is widely added to foods such as milk, it has additionally come into common practice in the

United States to promote vitamin D supplementation during pregnancy and infancy, which may thus produce benefits; effects should be monitored.

SALIVARY STIMULANTS

Currently, no clinical studies known to these authors have evaluated the effects of medications that stimulate salivary production against dental caries. Although saliva provides a natural defense against caries disease, and the most dramatic severity of disease occurs when saliva flow is severely decreased (xerostomia), no clinical trials have been performed to evaluate the possibility of protective effects against caries by muscarinic agents in patients with xerostomia. Xerostomia is a common, unintended side effect of many drugs with anticholinergic effects, or of radiation therapy, and Sjogren's disease. Of course, these studies would have to weigh the incidence of caries lesions, as manifested in the long term, versus the acute manifestations of the cholinergic (muscarinic) agent—desired salivation, lacrimation, perspiration, intestinal cramping, and defecation, and potentially bradycardia that are characteristic responses to muscarinic drugs.

SEALANTS FOR CARIES ARREST

In the pediatric chapter of *Pathology of the Hard Tissues of the Teeth*, Black instructs "Leave the decayed material in the dentin where it is," when describing interproximal disking and the use of silver nitrate to treat caries.[111] Many infections resolve with the use of antibiotics, which do not kill nor remove every causative microbe; rather, they tip the balance in favor of the host response and, when properly selected, to preferential survival of benign indigenous bacteria. Similarly, treating caries lesions by sealing them to remove access to host dietary nutrients or further insult tips the balance in favor of the host response. This is not new. Even the cautious American Dental Association Council on Scientific Affairs states that, "sealants can prevent the progression of early noncavitated carious lesions."[69] The goodness of the seal is the important factor. The abilities of the odontoblasts to specifically sense and secrete antimicrobial peptides that kill cariogenic bacteria, and to keep inflammation away from the inner pulp, seem to have been overlooked.[112] As well, reactionary dentin (tertiary) forms under slowed or arrested lesions, serving to distance the pulp from active microbes. Thus, most caries lesions should simply be sealed rather than excavated.

In the Hall technique, discussed elsewhere in this article, caries lesions are sealed with a pre-formed stainless steel or acrylic strip crown and glass ionomer luting cement; this is the single-most effective caries lesion treatment in primary teeth besides extraction.[113] The *Journal of the American Dental Association* has published studies for decades that demonstrate the long-term clinical and microbiological success of sealing in caries lesions that progress well into the dentin.[114] Bacteria die when cut off from nutrients. A recent systematic review in the *Journal of Dental Research* reports fewer pulp exposures and symptoms with incomplete excavation: "incomplete lesion removal seems advantageous compared with complete excavation, especially in proximity to the pulp."[115] Leaving some bacteria in a tooth with no signs or symptoms of pulpal pathology is becoming the standard of care; this technique is used when sealing in initial lesions as recommended by the American Dental Association, although some bacteria are nearly always found in sound or affected dentin. Meanwhile, therapeutic sealants can be combined with chemotherapeutic interventions such as silver diamine fluoride or silver nitrate provide.[116] Sealing caries lesions simply requires a good seal, which in turn demands either circumferential contact with healthy enamel, or complete coverage as with the Hall technique.

ATRAUMATIC RESTORATIVE TREATMENT

Atraumatic restorative treatment is the simple operative procedure of partial lesion removal, focusing on developing clean margins, followed by placement of a high-viscosity glass ionomer cement. Neither advanced equipment nor electricity is needed. The treatment of single surface lesions is highly useful, and success in multiple surface lesions has higher failure rates.[117] The conceptual novelty with respect to traditional operative dentistry has motivated various US professional organizations to attempt to rename atraumatic restorative treatment as "scoop and fill glass ionomers" or "interim therapeutic restorations." However, the inventors of the technique and the World Health Organization already named this and recommended its use worldwide, 20 years ago.

HALL TECHNIQUE CROWNS FOR ARREST

The Hall technique for placing stainless steel crowns is shockingly easy and effective. An appropriately sized, preformed crown is selected and cemented using a glass ionomer cement, with neither excavation of the lesion nor other mechanical or chemical preparation. The presumed therapeutic mechanism is multiple: seal the tooth from the inflow of extrinsic nutrients in an attempt to deprive cariogenic bacteria of nutrients, and strengthen the caries-weakened dentin with fluoride and metal ions from the cement.

Evidence supporting the Hall technique includes a 5-year split-mouth randomized controlled trial in 132 children, which not only evaluated minor (need for retreatment) and major (infection) failures, but also personal factors such as treatment preference. This study even followed 73% of teeth to exfoliation.[113] Another similar randomized trial followed 148 children. Concerns raised about the possibility of low-quality restorations in the control group in the first clinical trial were addressed in the second trial, in which all restorations were performed or supervised by pediatric dentists.[118]

BEHAVIORAL INTERVENTIONS

Current guidance from the American Academy of Pediatric Dentistry[119] and other professional organizations states that toothbrushing of all dentate children should be performed twice daily with a fluoridated toothpaste and parents should use a "smear" of toothpaste to brush the teeth of a child less than 2 years of age. Despite that recommendation, there is no evidence for the effectiveness of dentist anticipatory guidance or counseling. Studies of this topic, although imperfect,[120] are beginning to appear in the literature.[121] Although fluoride toothpaste is effective in the primary dentition (as discussed elsewhere in this article), the results question whether the age 1 dental visit is an efficacious means of informing and guiding parent and child behavior.

Trials of traditional advice-based counseling have been neither promising nor rigorous.[122] A search of trials on the effect of dietary interventions, for example, alone or in combination with other behavioral interventions on dental caries of children identified 13 trials. Self-reported increases in fruit and vegetable consumption was reported, but no changes in sugar consumption nor hygiene were achieved. Limitations of the studies included not having an intense phase as well as a maintenance phase of the intervention to maintain change, a short follow-up, and not including caries as an outcome. Moreover, the trial designs not only underestimate the need to impart specific parenting skills required to improve self-efficacy of caregivers in child's oral hygiene or child's sugar-sweetened beverage intake, but also lack an environmental component designed to limit access to cariogenic foods.

A better approach to controlling the etiologic sugar consumption is governmental policy. Studies of Mexico's tax on sugar-sweetened beverages show a 10% decrease in nation-wide consumption after 2 years, and more than $1 billion in government income.[2] A similar tax in Berkeley, California, demonstrated a 10% decrease in sugar beverages, and a 16% increase in water consumption.[123] Similar system-wide interventions should be adopted throughout North America and elsewhere, and research should be done to monitor the effects on caries.

Many low-income parents have difficulty acting on health recommendations and in following through with intentions to attend classes and clinics.[124] An intervention that involves parents in identifying their needs and helps them to overcome barriers to act on their needs is necessary. Traditional health education is insufficient to change parental behavior in at-risk populations. Health education in dental and medical settings is frequently an attempt to persuade. What seems to be a convincing line of reasoning to the dental or medical professional falls on deaf ears or results in a reluctance to change. Patients have reservations about "being told what to do," especially by a stranger.[125] More fundamental is the possibility that direct persuasion, whatever the degree of a patient's readiness to change, pushes the patient into a defensive position. Although health education has not been successful, there have been promising results using motivational interviewing. For example, Harrison and Wong[126] reported that children whose mothers received at least 2 counseling sessions using motivational interviewing regarding children's oral health needs and disease prevention had significantly less tooth decay than children in a comparison group. The motivational approach featured one-on-one counseling by a lay worker, personalization of recommendations, and telephone follow-up with the mothers. An experimental study by Weinstein and colleagues compared a brief counseling intervention, again using motivational interviewing, with traditional oral health education to reduce tooth decay in a sample of 240 high-risk infants, 6 to 18 months of age. A 50% reduction in tooth decay was associated with the motivational interviewing intervention.[127–129]

Motivational interviewing is a client-centered yet directive counseling approach. The conceptual basis is founded in the theory and research on self-regulation. Self-regulation models view individuals as active participants in reducing gaps between their perceived current status and immediate and long-term goals; health and illness behaviors are the result of the individual's representation of health threats and perceptions of the relevance of actions for managing or controlling these threats. The intervention approach that follows from the theory builds on client-centered counseling skills. It differs from traditional client-centered counseling in that the skills (ie, open-ended questioning, affirmations and the reinforcement of self-efficacy, reflective listening, and summarizing) are used in a highly directive manner that moves clients toward self-examination and awareness of the problem, and to understand how their current behavior is at odds with their desired goal. Motivational interviewing uses the stages of change model to understand the process of change and select specific strategies to move clients from a stage of inaction to action.

Case management is the facilitation, coordination, and monitoring of services, the purpose of which is to provide individuals with the ability to engage in actions to better their health. Case management helps to identify barriers that may preclude or interfere with client actions, helps to develop strategies to overcome these barriers, and at times provides advocacy for clients. In recent years, dental case management for families and children with low incomes was found to enhance dentist participation in Medicaid, and the use of dental services and result in increased oral health literacy.[130] Other studies have used case management to integrate dental and medical care[131] and to overcome barriers to accessing dental school services.[132]

AN AGE-GUIDED MODEL FOR DENTAL PUBLIC HEALTH

Assembling this article into an actionable recommendation for controlling dental caries using currently available materials is straightforward. Centralized approaches should include fluoridating the water and distributing fluoride toothpaste. Scalable, hands-on approaches should include the application of povidone iodine and fluoride varnish to high-risk children with increased frequency at younger ages, silver diamine fluoride to all caries lesions, and glass ionomer cement to seal cavitation with circumferential coronal tooth structure (the combination of silver diamine fluoride and glass ionomer cement should be encouraged). When lesions in primary teeth are large, the Hall technique should be used. These hands-on approaches should be delivered in the field by hygienists, therapists, or assistants, where patients frequent, namely, WICs, Head Starts, schools, Planned Parenthood, and long-term care facilities. The target populations are young children before 3 years of age and those 6 to 8 years of age; pregnant women; and those who are older. Older caregivers of young children should be sought with pick-up and drop-off to child day programs. School supervised brushing programs should be widely implemented at young ages, with a "spit not rinse" approach starting at 8 years of age. Xylitol gum should be given to new mothers through WICs for at least 1 year when the child is ages 3 to 15 months, and similarly to older caries active caregivers. Vitamin D levels should be surveyed regionally during pregnancy and infancy and supplemented accordingly. Finally, assessment of the time of initial *S mutans* colonization and the time of first apparent lesions for the target population of each public health unit should be done to inform the selection and timing of interventions.

The mainstay of caries prevention continues to be fluoride and control of sugar exposure, but metal ions, antiseptics, polyols, and vitamins may contribute as well. The mechanistic bases of protection are clear, in most cases, and comprehensive: fluorides increase the resilience of the tooth; reducing sugar exposure affects the cariogenic flora and acid production in the dental plaque; xylitol, silver, and iodine decrease the load of *S mutans*; and xylitol decreases transmission of *S mutans*. These interventions are appropriate to address the life events, during which people are most susceptible to experiencing caries lesions and passing down the infection.

REFERENCES

1. Kearns CE, Glantz SA, Schmidt LA. Sugar industry influence on the scientific agenda of the National Institute of Dental Research's 1971 National Caries Program: a historical analysis of internal documents. Capewell S, ed. PLoS Med 2015;12(3):e1001798.
2. Colchero MA, Rivera-Dommarco J, Popkin BM, et al. In Mexico, evidence of sustained consumer response two years after implementing a sugar-sweetened beverage tax. Health Aff (Millwood) 2017;36(3):564–71.
3. Sheiham A. Dental caries affects body weight, growth and quality of life in preschool children. Br Dent J 2006;201(10):625–6.
4. Nelson O, Mandelaris J, Ferretti O, et al. School screening and parental reminders in increasing dental care for children in need: a retrospective cohort study. J Public Health Dent 2012;72(1):45–52.
5. Köhler B, Andréen I. Influence of caries-preventive measures in mothers on cariogenic bacteria and caries experience in their children. Arch Oral Biol 1994; 39(10):907–11.
6. Thorild I, Lindau B, Twetman S. Caries in 4-year-old children after maternal chewing of gums containing combinations of xylitol, sorbitol, chlorhexidine and fluoride. Eur Arch Paediatr Dent 2006;7(4):241–5.

7. Alamoudi NM, Hanno AG, Almushayt AS, et al. Early prevention of childhood caries with maternal xylitol consumption. Saudi Med J 2014;35(6):592–7.
8. Isokangas P, Söderling E, Pienihäkkinen K, et al. Occurrence of dental decay in children after maternal consumption of xylitol chewing gum, a follow-up from 0 to 5 years of age. J Dent Res 2000;79(11):1885–9.
9. Milgrom P, Riedy CA, Weinstein P, et al. Dental caries and its relationship to bacterial infection, hypoplasia, diet, and oral hygiene in 6- to 36-month-old children. Community Dent Oral Epidemiol 2000;28(4):295–306.
10. Carlos JP, Gittelsohn AM. Longitudinal studies of the natural history of caries—II. Arch Oral Biol 1965;10(5):739–51.
11. Li Y, Wang W. Predicting caries in permanent teeth from caries in primary teeth: an eight-year cohort study. J Dent Res 2002;81(8):561–6.
12. Heller KE, Eklund SA, Pittman J, et al. Associations between dental treatment in the primary and permanent dentitions using insurance claims data. Pediatr Dent 2000;22(6):469–74.
13. Grembowski D, Milgrom PM. Increasing access to dental care for Medicaid preschool children: the Access to Baby and Child Dentistry (ABCD) program. Public Health Rep 2000;115(5):448–59.
14. Anusavice KJ. Present and future approaches for the control of caries. J Dent Educ 2005;69(5):538–54.
15. Twetman S, Dhar V. Evidence of effectiveness of current therapies to prevent and treat early childhood caries. Pediatr Dent 2015;37(3):246–53.
16. Gustafsson BE, Quensel CE, Lanke LS, et al. The Vipeholm Dental Caries Study; the effect of different levels of carbohydrate intake on caries activity in 436 individuals observed for five years. Acta Odontol Scand 1954;11(3–4):232–64.
17. Weiss RL, Trithart AH. Between-meal eating habits and dental caries experience in preschool children. Am J Public Health Nations Health 1960;50(8):1097–104.
18. Newbrun E, Hoover C, Mettraux G, et al. Comparison of dietary habits and dental health of subjects with hereditary fructose intolerance and control subjects. J Am Dent Assoc 1980;101(4):619–26.
19. van Houte J, Duchin S. Streptococcus mutans in the mouths of children with congenital sucrase deficiency. Arch Oral Biol 1975;20(11):771–3.
20. Paglia L. Does breastfeeding increase risk of early childhood caries? Eur J Paediatr Dent 2015;16(3):173.
21. Axelsson P, Kristoffersson K, Karlsson R, et al. A 30-month longitudinal study of the effects of some oral hygiene measures on Streptococcus mutans and approximal dental caries. J Dent Res 1987;66(3):761–5.
22. Marinho VCC, Worthington HV, Walsh T, et al. Fluoride varnishes for preventing dental caries in children and adolescents. Worthington HV, ed. Cochrane Database Syst Rev 2013;(7):CD002279.
23. Milgrom P, Taves DM, Kim AS, et al. Pharmacokinetics of fluoride in toddlers after application of 5% sodium fluoride dental varnish. Pediatrics 2014;134(3):e870–4.
24. Jiang EM, Lo EC-M, Chu C-H, et al. Prevention of early childhood caries (ECC) through parental toothbrushing training and fluoride varnish application: a 24-month randomized controlled trial. J Dent 2014;42(12):1543–50.
25. Agouropoulos A, Twetman S, Pandis N, et al. Caries-preventive effectiveness of fluoride varnish as adjunct to oral health promotion and supervised tooth brushing in preschool children: a double-blind randomized controlled trial. J Dent 2014;42(10):1277–83.

26. Oliveira BH, Salazar M, Carvalho DM, et al. Biannual fluoride varnish applications and caries incidence in preschoolers: a 24-month follow-up randomized placebo-controlled clinical trial. Caries Res 2014;48(3):228–36.

27. Memarpour M, Fakhraei E, Dadaein S, et al. Efficacy of fluoride varnish and casein phosphopeptide-amorphous calcium phosphate for remineralization of primary teeth: a randomized clinical trial. Med Princ Pract 2015;24(3):231–7.

28. Lawrence HP, Binguis D, Douglas J, et al. A 2-year community-randomized controlled trial of fluoride varnish to prevent early childhood caries in Aboriginal children. Community Dent Oral Epidemiol 2008;36(6):503–16.

29. Anderson M, Dahllöf G, Twetman S, et al. Effectiveness of early preventive intervention with semiannual fluoride varnish application in toddlers living in high-risk areas: a stratified cluster-randomized controlled trial. Caries Res 2016;50(1):17–23.

30. Ramos-Gomez FJ, Gansky SA, Featherstone JDB, et al. Mother and youth access (MAYA) maternal chlorhexidine, counselling and paediatric fluoride varnish randomized clinical trial to prevent early childhood caries. Int J Paediatr Dent 2012;22(3):169–79.

31. Tickle M, O'Neill C, Donaldson M, et al. A randomised controlled trial to measure the effects and costs of a dental caries prevention regime for young children attending primary care dental services: the Northern Ireland Caries Prevention In Practice (NIC-PIP) trial. Health Technol Assess 2016;20(71):1–96.

32. Slade GD, Bailie RS, Roberts-Thomson K, et al. Effect of health promotion and fluoride varnish on dental caries among Australian Aboriginal children: results from a community-randomized controlled trial. Community Dent Oral Epidemiol 2011;39(1):29–43.

33. Dehailan Al L, Lippert F, González-Cabezas C, et al. Fluoride concentration in saliva and biofilm fluid following the application of three fluoride varnishes. J Dent 2017;60:87–93.

34. Lopez L, Berkowitz R, Spiekerman C, et al. Topical antimicrobial therapy in the prevention of early childhood caries: a follow-up report. Pediatr Dent 2002;24(3):204–6.

35. Milgrom PM, Tut OK, Mancl LA. Topical iodine and fluoride varnish effectiveness in the primary dentition: a quasi-experimental study. J Dent Child (Chic) 2011;78(3):143–7.

36. Tubert-Jeannin S, Auclair C, Amsallem E, et al. Fluoride supplements (tablets, drops, lozenges or chewing gums) for preventing dental caries in children. Tubert-Jeannin S, ed. Cochrane Database Syst Rev 2011;(12):CD007592.

37. Harding MA, O'Mullane DM. Water fluoridation and oral health. Acta Med Acad 2013;42(2):131–9.

38. Iheozor-Ejiofor Z, Worthington HV, Walsh T, et al. Water fluoridation for the prevention of dental caries. Glenny A-M, ed. Cochrane Database Syst Rev 2015;(6):CD010856.

39. Marthaler TM. Salt fluoridation and oral health. Acta Med Acad 2013;42(2):140–55.

40. Bánóczy J, Rugg-Gunn A, Woodward M. Milk fluoridation for the prevention of dental caries. Acta Med Acad 2013;42(2):156–67.

41. Yeung CA, Chong LY, Glenny A-M. Fluoridated milk for preventing dental caries. Yeung CA, ed. Cochrane Database Syst Rev 2015;(9):CD003876.

42. Walsh T, Worthington HV, Glenny A-M, et al. Fluoride toothpastes of different concentrations for preventing dental caries in children and adolescents. Walsh T, ed. Cochrane Database Syst Rev 2010;(1):CD007868.

43. Ellwood RP, Davies GM, Worthington HV, et al. Relationship between area deprivation and the anticaries benefit of an oral health programme providing free

fluoride toothpaste to young children. Community Dent Oral Epidemiol 2004; 32(3):159–65.

44. Wright JT, Hanson N, Ristic H, et al. Fluoride toothpaste efficacy and safety in children younger than 6 years: a systematic review. J Am Dent Assoc 2014; 145(2):182–9.

45. Wong MC, Glenny A-M, Tsang BW, et al. Topical fluoride as a cause of dental fluorosis in children. Wong MC, ed. Cochrane Database Syst Rev 2010;(1):CD007693.

46. Aimée NR, van Wijk AJ, Maltz M, et al. Dental caries, fluorosis, oral health determinants, and quality of life in adolescents. Clin Oral Investig 2017;21(5):1811–20.

47. Marinho VCC, Higgins JPT, Logan S, et al. Topical fluoride (toothpastes, mouthrinses, gels or varnishes) for preventing dental caries in children and adolescents. Marinho VC, ed. Cochrane Database Syst Rev 2003;(4):CD002782.

48. Marinho VCC, Chong LY, Worthington HV, et al. Fluoride mouthrinses for preventing dental caries in children and adolescents. Marinho VC, ed. Cochrane Database Syst Rev 2016;(7):CD002284.

49. Marinho VCC, Higgins JPT, Sheiham A, et al. One topical fluoride (toothpastes, or mouthrinses, or gels, or varnishes) versus another for preventing dental caries in children and adolescents. Marinho VC, ed. Cochrane Database Syst Rev 2004;(1):CD002780.

50. Horst JA, Ellenikiotis H, Milgrom PL. UCSF protocol for caries arrest using silver diamine fluoride: rationale, indications and consent. J Calif Dent Assoc 2016; 44(1):16–28.

51. Mei ML, Chu C-H, Lo EC-M, et al. Fluoride and silver concentrations of silver diammine fluoride solutions for dental use. Int J Paediatr Dent 2013;23(4): 279–85.

52. Mei ML, Li Q-L, Chu C-H, et al. Antibacterial effects of silver diamine fluoride on multi-species cariogenic biofilm on caries. Ann Clin Microbiol Antimicrob 2013; 12:4.

53. Mei ML, Chu C-H, Low K-H, et al. Caries arresting effect of silver diamine fluoride on dentine carious lesion with S. mutans and L. acidophilus dual-species cariogenic biofilm. Med Oral Patol Oral Cir Bucal 2013;18(6):e824–31.

54. Knight GM, McIntyre JM, Craig GG, et al. Inability to form a biofilm of Streptococcus mutans on silver fluoride- and potassium iodide-treated demineralized dentin. Quintessence Int 2009;40(2):155–61.

55. Llodra JC, Rodriguez A, Ferrer B, et al. Efficacy of silver diamine fluoride for caries reduction in primary teeth and first permanent molars of schoolchildren: 36-month clinical trial. J Dent Res 2005;84(8):721–4.

56. Zhi QH, Lo EC-M, Lin HC. Randomized clinical trial on effectiveness of silver diamine fluoride and glass ionomer in arresting dentine caries in preschool children. J Dent 2012;40(11):962–7.

57. Yee R, Holmgren C, Mulder J, et al. Efficacy of silver diamine fluoride for arresting caries treatment. J Dent Res 2009;88(7):644–7.

58. Fung MHT, Duangthip D, Wong MCM, et al. Arresting dentine caries with different concentration and periodicity of silver diamine fluoride. JDR Clin Trans Res 2016;1(2):143–52.

59. Chu CH, Lo ECM, Lin HC. Effectiveness of silver diamine fluoride and sodium fluoride varnish in arresting dentin caries in Chinese pre-school children. J Dent Res 2002;81(11):767–70.

60. Tan HP, Lo ECM, Dyson JE, et al. A randomized trial on root caries prevention in elders. J Dent Res 2010;89(10):1086–90.

61. Liu BY, Lo ECM, Li CMT. Effect of silver and fluoride ions on enamel demineralization: a quantitative study using micro-computed tomography. Aust Dent J 2012;57(1):65–70.

62. Crystal YO, Janal MN, Hamilton DS, et al. Parental perceptions and acceptance of silver diamine fluoride staining. J Am Dent Assoc 2017;148(7):510–8.e4.

63. Chu CH, Lo ECM. Microhardness of dentine in primary teeth after topical fluoride applications. J Dent 2008;36(6):387–91.

64. Cueto EI, Buonocore MG. Sealing of pits and fissures with an adhesive resin: its use in caries prevention. J Am Dent Assoc 1967;75(1):121–8.

65. Liu BY, Lo ECM, Chu CH, et al. Randomized trial on fluorides and sealants for fissure caries prevention. J Dent Res 2012;91(8):753–8.

66. Tagliaferro EPDS, Pardi V, Ambrosano GMB, et al. Occlusal caries prevention in high and low risk schoolchildren. A clinical trial. Am J Dent 2011;24(2):109–14.

67. Chestnutt IG, Hutchings S, Playle R, et al. Seal or Varnish? A randomised controlled trial to determine the relative cost and effectiveness of pit and fissure sealant and fluoride varnish in preventing dental decay. Health Technol Assess 2017;21(21):1–256.

68. Sun BC, Chi DL, Schwarz E, et al. Emergency department visits for nontraumatic dental problems: a mixed-methods study. Am J Public Health 2015;105(5): 947–55.

69. Wright JT, Crall JJ, Fontana M, et al. Evidence-based clinical practice guideline for the use of pit-and-fissure sealants: a report of the American Dental Association and the American Academy of Pediatric Dentistry. J Am Dent Assoc 2016;147(8):672–82.e12.

70. Mickenautsch S, Yengopal V. Caries-preventive effect of high-viscosity glass ionomer and resin-based fissure sealants on permanent teeth: a systematic review of clinical trials. Gándara E, ed. PLoS One 2016;11(1):e0146512.

71. Cagetti MG, Carta G, Cocco F, et al. Effect of fluoridated sealants on adjacent tooth surfaces: a 30-mo randomized clinical trial. J Dent Res 2014; 93(7 Suppl):59S–65S.

72. Trahan L. Xylitol: a review of its action on mutans streptococci and dental plaque–its clinical significance. Int Dent J 1995;45(1 Suppl 1):77–92.

73. Scheinin A, Mäkinen KK. Turku sugar studies. An overview. Acta Odontol Scand 1976;34(6):405–8.

74. Scheinin A, Mäkinen KK, Tammisalo E, et al. Turku sugar studies XVIII. Incidence of dental caries in relation to 1-year consumption of xylitol chewing gum. Acta Odontol Scand 1975;33(5):269–78.

75. Dawes C. Xylitol as caries prevention? Caries Res 2010;44(2):170 [author reply: 170].

76. Mäkinen KK, Bennett CA, Hujoel PP, et al. Xylitol chewing gums and caries rates: a 40-month cohort study. J Dent Res 1995;74(12):1904–13.

77. Sintes JL, Elías-Boneta A, Stewart B, et al. Anticaries efficacy of a sodium monofluorophosphate dentifrice containing xylitol in a dicalcium phosphate dihydrate base. A 30-month caries clinical study in Costa Rica. Am J Dent 2002;15(4): 215–9.

78. Sintes JL, Escalante C, Stewart B, et al. Enhanced anticaries efficacy of a 0.243% sodium fluoride/10% xylitol/silica dentifrice: 3-year clinical results. Am J Dent 1995;8(5):231–5.

79. Chi DL, Tut O, Milgrom P. Cluster-randomized xylitol toothpaste trial for early childhood caries prevention. J Dent Child (Chic) 2014;81(1):27–32.

80. Ritter AV, Bader JD, Leo MC, et al. Tooth-surface-specific effects of xylitol: randomized trial roaulto. J Dent Res 2013;92(6):512–7

81. Slee AM, Tanzer JM. The repressible metabolism of sorbitol (D-glucitol) by intact cells of the oral plaque-forming bacterium Streptococcus mutans. Arch Oral Biol 1983;28(9):839–45.

82. Birkhed D, Edwardsson S, Ahldén M-L, et al. Effects of 3 months frequent consumption of hydrogenated starch hydrolysate (Lycasin®), maltitol, sorbitol and xylitol on human dental plaque. Acta Odontol Scand 2009;37(2):103–15.

83. de Cock P. Erythritol. In: O'Donnell K, Kearsley M, editors. Sweeteners and sugar alternatives in food technology (2nd edition). Oxford (United Kingdom): Wiley-Blackwell; 2012. p. 215–42.

84. Mäkinen KK, Isotupa KP, Kivilompolo T, et al. Comparison of erythritol and xylitol saliva stimulants in the control of dental plaque and mutans streptococci. Caries Res 2001;35(2):129–35.

85. Lenkkeri A-MH, Pienihäkkinen K, Hurme S, et al. The caries-preventive effect of xylitol/maltitol and erythritol/maltitol lozenges: results of a double-blinded, cluster-randomized clinical trial in an area of natural fluoridation. Int J Paediatr Dent 2012;22(3):180–90.

86. Joo JE, Jung IH, Cho KS, et al. Low cariogenicity of maltosyl-erythritol, major transglycosylation product of erythritol, by Bacillus stearothemophilus maltogenic amylase. J Microbiol Biotech 2003;13:815–8.

87. Honkala S, Runnel R, Saag M, et al. Effect of erythritol and xylitol on dental caries prevention in children. Caries Res 2014;48(5):482–90.

88. Imfeld T. Efficacy of sweeteners and sugar substitutes in caries prevention. Caries Res 1993;27(Suppl 1):50–5.

89. Imfeld TN. Identification of low caries risk dietary components. Monogr Oral Sci 1983;11:1–198.

90. Handelman SL, Mills JR, Hawes RR. Caries incidence in subjects receiving long term antibiotic therapy. J Oral Ther Pharmacol 1966;2(5):338–45.

91. Zickert I, Emilson CG, Krasse B. Effect of caries preventive measures in children highly infected with the bacterium Streptococcus mutans. Arch Oral Biol 1982; 27(10):861–8.

92. Hildebrandt GH, Sparks BS. Maintaining mutans streptococci suppression with xylitol chewing gum. J Am Dent Assoc 2000;131(7):909–16.

93. Slot DE, Vaandrager NC, Van Loveren C, et al. The effect of chlorhexidine varnish on root caries: a systematic review. Caries Res 2011;45(2):162–73.

94. Walsh T, Oliveira-Neto JM, Moore D. Chlorhexidine treatment for the prevention of dental caries in children and adolescents. Walsh T, ed. Cochrane Database Syst Rev 2015;(4):CD008457.

95. Papas AS, Vollmer WM, Gullion CM, et al. Efficacy of chlorhexidine varnish for the prevention of adult caries: a randomized trial. J Dent Res 2012;91(2):150–5.

96. Tanzer JM, Livingston J, Thompson AM. The microbiology of primary dental caries in humans. J Dent Educ 2001;65(10):1028–37.

97. Gisselsson H, Birkhed D, Björn AL. Effect of a 3-year professional flossing program with chlorhexidine gel on approximal caries and cost of treatment in preschool children. Caries Res 1994;28(5):394–9.

98. Zhan L, Featherstone JDB, Gansky SA, et al. Antibacterial treatment needed for severe early childhood caries. J Public Health Dent 2006;66(3):174–9.

99. Berkowitz RJ, Amante A, Kopycka-Kedzierawski DT, et al. Dental caries recurrence following clinical treatment for severe early childhood caries. Pediatr Dent 2011;33(7):510–4.

100. Tut OK, Milgrom PM. Topical iodine and fluoride varnish combined is more effective than fluoride varnish alone for protecting erupting first permanent molars: a retrospective cohort study. J Public Health Dent 2010;70(3):249–52.

101. Li X, Zhong Y, Jiang X, et al. Randomized clinical trial of the efficacy of dentifrices containing 1.5% arginine, an insoluble calcium compound and 1450 ppm fluoride over two years. J Clin Dent 2015;26(1):7–12.

102. Acevedo AM, Machado C, Rivera LE, et al. The inhibitory effect of an arginine bicarbonate/calcium carbonate CaviStat-containing dentifrice on the development of dental caries in Venezuelan school children. J Clin Dent 2005;16(3): 63–70.

103. Kraivaphan P, Amornchat C, Triratana T, et al. Two-year caries clinical study of the efficacy of novel dentifrices containing 1.5% arginine, an insoluble calcium compound and 1,450 ppm fluoride. Caries Res 2013;47(6):582–90.

104. Hu DY, Yin W, Li X, et al. A clinical investigation of the efficacy of a dentifrice containing 1.5% arginine and 1450 ppm fluoride, as sodium monofluorophosphate in a calcium base, on primary root caries. J Clin Dent 2013;24(Spec no A): A23–31.

105. Souza MLR, Cury JA, Tenuta LMA, et al. Comparing the efficacy of a dentifrice containing 1.5% arginine and 1450 ppm fluoride to a dentifrice containing 1450 ppm fluoride alone in the management of primary root caries. J Dent 2013; 41(Suppl 2):S35–41.

106. Nascimento MM, Browngardt C, Xiaohui X, et al. The effect of arginine on oral biofilm communities. Mol Oral Microbiol 2014;29(1):45–54.

107. Hujoel PP. Vitamin D and dental caries in controlled clinical trials: systematic review and meta-analysis. Nutr Rev 2013;71(2):88–97.

108. Schroth RJ, Lavelle C, Tate R, et al. Prenatal vitamin D and dental caries in infants. Pediatrics 2014;133(5):e1277–84.

109. Schroth RJ, Rabbani R, Loewen G, et al. Vitamin D and dental caries in children. J Dent Res 2016;95(2):173–9.

110. Herzog K, Scott JM, Hujoel P, et al. Association of vitamin D and dental caries in children: findings from the National Health and Nutrition Examination Survey, 2005-2006. J Am Dent Assoc 2016;147(6):413–20.

111. Black GV. The pathology of the hard tissues of the teeth, vol. 1. Chicago: Medico-Dental Publishing Company; 1908.

112. Horst OV, Horst JA, Samudrala R, et al. Caries induced cytokine network in the odontoblast layer of human teeth. BMC Immunol 2011;12:9.

113. Innes N, Stewart M, Souster G, et al. The hall technique; retrospective case-note follow-up of 5-year RCT. Br Dent J 2015;219(8):395–400.

114. Mertz-Fairhurst EJ, Curtis JW, Ergle JW, et al. Ultraconservative and cariostatic sealed restorations: results at year 10. J Am Dent Assoc 1998;129(1):55–66.

115. Schwendicke F, Dörfer CE, Paris S. Incomplete caries removal: a systematic review and meta-analysis. J Dent Res 2013;92(4):306–14.

116. Horst J, Frachella JC, Duffin S. Response to letter to the editor. Pediatr Dent 2016;38(7):462–3.

117. de Amorim RG, Leal SC, Frencken JE. Survival of atraumatic restorative treatment (ART) sealants and restorations: a meta-analysis. Clin Oral Investig 2012;16(2):429–41.

118. Santamaria RM, Innes NPT, Machiulskiene V, et al. Caries management strategies for primary molars: 1-yr randomized control trial results. J Dent Res 2014;93(11):1062–9.

119. American Academy of Pediatric Dentistry. Clinical Affairs Committee–Infant Oral Health Subcommittee. Guideline on infant oral health care. Pediatr Dent 2012; 34(5):e148–52.

120. Milgrom PM, Cunha-Cruz J. Are tooth decay prevention visits in primary care before age 2 years effective? JAMA Pediatr 2017;171(4):321–2.

121. Blackburn J, Morrisey MA, Sen B. Outcomes associated with early preventive dental care among medicaid-enrolled children in Alabama. JAMA Pediatr 2017;171(4):335–41.

122. Harris R, Gamboa A, Dailey Y, et al. One-to-one dietary interventions undertaken in a dental setting to change dietary behaviour. Harris R, ed. Cochrane Database Syst Rev 2012;(3):CD006540.

123. Silver LD, Ng SW, Ryan-Ibarra S, et al. Changes in prices, sales, consumer spending, and beverage consumption one year after a tax on sugar-sweetened beverages in Berkeley, California, US: a before-and-after study. Langenberg C, ed. PLoS Med 2017;14(4):e1002283.

124. Mah JWT, Johnston C. Parental social cognitions: considerations in the acceptability of and engagement in behavioral parent training. Clin Child Fam Psychol Rev 2008;11(4):218–36.

125. Stott NC, Pill RM. 'Advise yes, dictate no'. Patients' views on health promotion in the consultation. Fam Pract 1990;7(2):125–31.

126. Harrison RL, Wong T. An oral health promotion program for an urban minority population of preschool children. Community Dent Oral Epidemiol 2003;31(5): 392–9.

127. Harrison R, Benton T, Everson-Stewart S, et al. Effect of motivational interviewing on rates of early childhood caries: a randomized trial. Pediatr Dent 2007;29(1): 16–22.

128. Weinstein P, Harrison R, Benton T. Motivating mothers to prevent caries: confirming the beneficial effect of counseling. J Am Dent Assoc 2006;137(6):789–93.

129. Weinstein P, Harrison R, Benton T. Motivating parents to prevent caries in their young children: one-year findings. J Am Dent Assoc 2004;135(6):731–8.

130. Greenberg BJS, Kumar JV, Stevenson H. Dental case management: increasing access to oral health care for families and children with low incomes. J Am Dent Assoc 2008;139(8):1114–21.

131. Wysen KH, Hennessy PM, Lieberman MI, et al. Kids get care: integrating preventive dental and medical care using a public health case management model. J Dent Educ 2004;68(5):522–30.

132. Zittel-Palamara K, Fabiano JA, Davis EL, et al. Improving patient retention and access to oral health care: the CARES program. J Dent Educ 2005;69(8):912–8.

133. Amin MS, Harrison RL, Benton TS, et al. Effect of povidone-iodine on Streptococcus mutans in children with extensive dental caries. Pediatr Dent 2004; 26(1):5–10.

134. Simratvir M, Singh N, Chopra S, et al. Efficacy of 10% Povidone Iodine in children affected with early childhood caries: an in vivo study. J Clin Pediatr Dent 2010;34(3):233–8.

135. Xu X, Li JY, Zhou XD, et al. Randomized controlled clinical trial on the evaluation of bacteriostatic and cariostatic effects of a novel povidone-iodine/fluoride foam in children with high caries risk. Quintessence Int 2009;40(3):215–23.

Infant Oral Health
An Emerging Dental Public Health Measure

Paul S. Casamassimo, DDS, MS[a],*, Kimberly Hammersmith, DDS, MPH, MS[b],
Erin L. Gross, DDS, PhD, MS[a], Homa Amini, DDS, MS, MPH[b]

KEYWORDS

- Infant oral health • Well-child care • Pediatric dentistry • Dental public health
- Prevention

KEY POINTS

- A child's first oral health visit should occur by 1 year of age to maximize preventive potential of fluorides, health literacy, and dietary modification. Caries increases with age so early intervention can reduce caries incidence, as evidenced by several studies.
- Interprofessional care optimizes the likelihood that a child will receive preventive intervention and also referral to a dental home. Oral health when integrated into primary medical care can result in improved outcomes for children. A simple message of fluoride adequacy, dietary control of bottle use and sweet intake, oral hygiene, and regular dental visits crosses professional barriers.
- Primary preventive oral care is preferable to treatment if at all possible. Recent concerns about the risks of general anesthesia and sedation and the continuing problem of pain from early childhood caries make prevention of caries preferable to a larger provider workforce.

INTRODUCTION

Infant oral health (IOH) is a well-child practice advocated for many years, but remains slow to gain universal acceptance among medical and dental professionals.[1] Simply defined, IOH is a child's first visit to a dentist between 6 and 12 months of age for examination and a dental caries risk assessment. Parents also receive preventive instruction, establish a dentist-family relationship (the dental home), and in most cases, have the health professional apply fluoride varnish to the child's primary teeth. IOH is advocated by the American Academy of Pediatric Dentistry (AAPD), the American Dental Association, and the American Academy of Pediatrics, among major

Disclosure Statement: The authors have nothing to disclose.
[a] The Ohio State University College of Dentistry, Nationwide Children's Hospital, 305 West 12th Avenue, Columbus, OH 43210, USA; [b] The Ohio State University College of Dentistry, Nationwide Children's Hospital, 700 Children's Drive, Columbus, OH 43205, USA
* Corresponding author.
E-mail address: casamassimo.1@osu.edu

health organizations.[1-3] IOH may be the purview of the primary care medical provider (PCP) when referral to a dentist is not possible. When viewed from a public health perspective, IOH serves a purpose of primary prevention parallel to the generally accepted practice of well-child visits by a PCP for developmental screening, immunizations, and anticipatory guidance. IOH is intended to prevent the initiation of dental caries, establish oral health literacy and good oral health behaviors in the family, and create the dental home relationship with a dentist for both recurring and urgent needs during the child's early life.[4]

The public health benefit of IOH in preventing early childhood caries (ECC) has yet to be realized but has immense potential to reduce the epidemic of ECC, a largely preventable childhood infectious disease with high human and societal costs. IOH will take a long time in public health practice to manifest benefits and must become part of the fabric of health supervision for that to happen. For several of the programs mentioned in this article, available data are limited to percentages of children receiving fluoride varnish, without accounting of caries reduction as an outcome. Ironically, the initial effect of large-scale IOH projects, rather than prevention, is to identify very young children already with disease and refer them to dental treatment. In a recent report by Bruen and colleagues[5] on the cost of general anesthesia, 2 states with a large penetration of IOH also had some of the highest costs for general anesthesia services to treat ECC. In the long term, with rigorous application of IOH in both medical and dental practice, a reduction in disease and its negative system and individual effects should soon be expected to be seen, although data are lacking because of its novelty and low penetration in practice to date.

SCIENCE AND RATIONALE FOR INFANT ORAL HEALTH

A major goal of IOH is to identify children at risk for ECC, so actions can be taken to prevent this disease. Initiation of ECC with establishment of infection can begin a lifelong propensity to new caries. The AAPD, among others, publishes a guideline on caries-risk assessment that considers biological factors, protective factors, and clinical findings to determine caries risk for each child.[6] Primary factors are the oral microbiome and the child's diet. ECC results when dietary sugars are metabolized by oral bacteria to acids that demineralize tooth structure. Bacterial communities associated with oral health are complex and, although they contain acid-producing species, can respond to sugar exposures and remain stable. However, when sugars are consumed more frequently, the increasingly acidic environment selects more acidogenic and aciduric species and the community shifts to become dominated by these species.[7] *Streptococcus mutans* (SM) is well established as a common acid producer in caries,[8] but other acid-producing species have also been associated with the disease.[9] SM is acquired by both vertical transmission (usually from the mother) and horizontal transmission and has been found in predentate infants.[10] Although oral bacteria and their acids are frequently listed among the causes of caries, a recent publication stressed that "sugars start the process" and criticized the common designation of caries as a multifactorial disease.[11] This review emphasized that without sugar, caries would not occur. IOH intervenes in this process in 2 ways: with dietary modification and institution of tooth cleaning, ideally for both child and primary caregiver. Going to bed with a bottle and frequently having sugary drinks or snacks between meals are risk factors for caries.[12] Maternal transmission and reinfection are possible and make maternal oral health important and a part of IOH in a public health setting.

During IOH visits, practitioners identify these factors and other behaviors that put the child at risk and develop individualized strategies that the family can use to prevent initiation and progression of disease. This interaction takes advantage of a heightened parental receptiveness and, with use of motivational interviewing techniques, can be an effective tool for behavioral change.[13]

Ultimately, the goal is to prevent ECC, which at this age causes pain and infection with their potential long-term effects and stress and costs for families, decreasing their quality of life.[14] Recent literature suggests that treatment under general anesthesia or deep sedation in very young children may be associated with long-term irreversible effects[15] and in itself is a reason to prevent caries in the infant and toddler age group. In addition, literature suggests that treating ECC with expensive restorations is not a cure for the disease; levels of caries pathogens are unchanged following restorative treatment.[16,17] In fact, recent work found that although the number of bacterial strains was reduced following restoration, dominant strains that were detected posttreatment were highly acidogenic strains of SM.[18]

Finally, the rationale for IOH includes beginning with the PCP as the dental home because children in the first years of life are far more likely to be seen by a physician than a dental professional. A well-functioning IOH system would initiate identification of oral health during well-child visits, referral to a dentist, and ideally, for young children already affected by dental caries, inclusion of a pediatric dentist as a source of treatment requiring advanced behavior guidance techniques such as sedation or general anesthesia.

OBSTACLES TO UNIVERSAL ACCEPTANCE OF INFANT ORAL HEALTH

Although well-child visits to a PCP are a staple of early health care for children, IOH has struggled to become integrated into either pediatric medical or general dental practice. In medical practice, the early well-child visit has remained static in time allotment at just under 20 minutes, yet PCPs are expected to address more than 50 policies containing 192 health directives.[19] The addition of oral health to an already overcrowded visit has usually occurred only when made a clinic or practice priority.[20] Many pediatricians view oral health as a far lower priority than many other pediatric health issues like obesity, behavior, safety, and mental health and prefer to have dentists address it with families. Lack of oral health education in medical training, lack of reimbursement for time spent, and untrained auxiliary staff round out reasons physicians have not embraced IOH in well-child care.[21]

In the dental community, a similar pattern of obstacles emerges, beginning with a lack of IOH training in dental school. Compounding dentists' lack of training is inadequate reimbursement by payers, disruption of practice patterns geared toward restoration and surgery, and a culture of practice unaccustomed to working with infants. General dentists do not see very young children and even today, only about half receive training in IOH.[22] Almost all pediatric dentists recently surveyed agreed with the age-1 dental visit policy and saw patients of this age for preventive visits,[23] and in another survey, half of responding pediatric dentists thought that general dentists should be seeing 1 year olds for preventive visits.[24] Surveys of general dentists have found that 42% of Connecticut general dentists,[25] and 45% of Virginia general dentists,[26] are caring for 0 to 2 year olds. However, the Virginia study found that only 5% of pediatricians and 12% of general dentists referred for the first dental visit by 1 year of age.[26]

When dentists and PCPs perform IOH, it is often in the context of an organized promotion, such as the Access to Baby and Child Dentistry (ABCD) program in Washington, the Into the Mouths of Babes (IMB) program in North Carolina, or the From the First Tooth program in the northeast (**Table 1**). State departments of health,

Table 1
Examples of infant oral health programs in medical and dental public health settings

Name of Program	Location	Provider	Description	Began	Outcomes
Access to Baby and Child Dentistry	Washington	Dentists	IOH training for dentists and pairs patients aged 0–6 with dentists for preventive care. ABCD providers receive enhanced fees	1999	Increased access to dental care for Medicaid-eligible children, 52% compared with 21% in 1999[44]
Into the Mouth of Babes	North Carolina	Physicians	Physicians trained in oral evaluation and risk assessment apply fluoride varnish up to 6 times before age 42 mo for Medicaid-eligible children	2004	Statewide decline in caries, reduction in gap between low- and higher-income families at community level[31]
From the First Tooth	Connecticut, Maine, Massachusetts, New Hampshire, Rhode Island, Vermont	Physicians	Physicians trained in oral evaluation and risk assessment apply fluoride varnish to children. Obstetricians trained to provide guidance to pregnant women[34]	2008	Multistate activity tied into primary care and in some states appearing on quality dashboards along with immunizations and other well-child measures
Dental Hygiene Co-Location Project	Colorado	Independent hygienists	Independent dental hygienists were located within medical practices, with dual-function examination rooms, and performed hygiene procedures. Pilot project consisted of 5 sites	2009	Full-time colocation better at shifting culture, increasing medical providers' oral health awareness and literacy. Lessons learned have influenced the Colorado Medica - Dental Integration Project[36]
Enhanced Oral Health Interventions in Primary Care/ Contra Costa Regional Medical Center	California	Physicians	Safety-net and academic partnership providing oral health information, screening, and referral during well-child examinations for children ages 1–5	2011	Physicians can effectively provide caries preventive services, enhanced knowledge of medical providers[40]

accountable care organizations, payers, or health coalitions may provide the impetus to address the above obstacles in a systematic fashion. The growing movement toward interprofessional care may also cause IOH to grow in acceptance, because roles and other critical factors shift to address patient needs across traditional boundaries. The presence of both medical and dental services in many Federally Qualified Health Centers has also enhanced the likelihood that a comprehensive care program for children includes IOH. **Table 1** describes the above and other programs on IOH that have been reported

EVIDENCE ONLY EMERGING ON BENEFITS OF INFANT ORAL HEALTH

As a public health measure, IOH is new, and its lack of penetration into health care practice makes evidence of its benefit limited. Longitudinal studies of both Medicaid-insured and privately insured children suggest a considerable cost savings associated with children who receive early dental visits compared with their peers who do not have a visit until later in childhood.[27–29] A more recent study, based on Medicaid claims data, found no difference among groups seen by PCPs, or not at all, based on services. The study did not account for patient variation, previous care, health literacy, or the level of ECC, so its utility in assessing IOH is very limited.[30] Another study found that cost-savings and difference in outcomes were negligible for children at lower risk of dental disease when comparing the first visits at age 3 and earlier.[31]

The long-term benefits of IOH remain to be demonstrated conclusively because of its current underutilization by both PCPs and dentists. Exposure to established and proven preventive techniques may remain the major source of justification for IOH for some time. The IMB program in North Carolina wherein physicians are trained to assess oral health of children and apply fluoride varnish has been shown to reduce caries; the reduction was larger when targeting higher-risk children.[32] IMB and the From the First Tooth Program, which operates in 5 northeastern states, have increased access for children to early preventive dental care by physicians.[33,34] The ABCD program of Washington State pairs Medicaid-insured children ages 0 to 6 with dentists to improve access to preventive care. The program has improved oral health awareness and increased preventive dental visits for both ABCD enrollees and non-ABCD enrollees.[35]

INFANT ORAL HEALTH AS A PUBLIC HEALTH TOOL

Beyond its attractiveness as a primary preventive tool, IOH fits into dental public health principles and practice. IOH also fits well into the goals of improved health for populations as described in the triple aims for health care in the United States, which are a better patient experience, improved health of the population, and lower cost. The following can be considered public health aspects of IOH:

1. Engagement of providers across health disciplines, offering more opportunities for high impact with minimal intervention;
2. Performance by multilevel personnel in several disciplines, keeping costs low as envisioned in the triple aims;
3. Primary prevention of disease, and secondarily, early identification of incipient disease, so lower cost of care;
4. Improved population health through health literacy and minimal interventions, such as fluoride varnish and motivational interviewing;

5. Improved health experience by reduction in dental disease and its consequences, as well as low-intensity treatment [14]

IOH is a relatively simple service, not necessitating the trappings of a dental office or clinic. Instrumentation is minimal, allowing its purveyance in almost any community or remote setting. Trained personnel, such as dental hygienists and expanded function dental assistants, at lower pay levels, can bring about positive outcomes with IOH making it cost-effective. A program in Colorado in which independent dental hygienists colocated into pediatric medical offices to perform basic preventive care proved this was even a feasible model of care.[36] Therapeutic interventions are largely with fluoride varnish contributing to its low cost. Even with the additions of silver diamine fluoride (SDF)[37] and interim therapeutic restorations[38] as the concept of minimally invasive pediatric dentistry grows, IOH remains attractive compared with other treatment approaches with greater risks to the child and costs to family or insurer, when it is not performed.

FINANCING INFANT ORAL HEALTH

One factor that impacts access to oral health care for infants and young children is availability of finances to cover the cost. In the United States, Medicaid is the largest publically funded insurance program that covers the cost of health care for low-income children, funded by a combination of federal and state dollars.[39] In 2015, Medicaid provided health coverage for 43% of US children, according to Congressional Budget Office estimates.[40] The income requirements for families for Medicaid coverage coincides with the high concentration of ECC in poor children, making Medicaid an ideal and necessary source of financing for IOH.

Medicaid's Early and Periodic Screening, Diagnosis, and Treatment (EPSDT) program that mandates comprehensive health care for children less than age 21 includes dental coverage for relief of pain and infections, restoration of teeth, and maintenance of dental health. Dental care for children is also subject to the "medical necessity" parameters, meaning benefits should include all services needed to address oral health conditions and each state should establish a periodicity schedule for dental services in line with recommended intervals set by standards of dental practice.[39,41] This requirement fits in with IOH, and over the decades since Medicaid's inception, states have adopted schedules that permit reimbursement for early dental intervention. The 2013 study by Hom and colleagues[41] revealed that all 50 states and the District of Columbia had a dental component to their EPSDT program. However, only 32 states and the District of Columbia had established a separate periodicity schedule. A majority (30 states) have adopted the AAPD periodicity guidelines, which establish frequency of clinical oral examination, caries risk assessment, topical fluoride application, anticipatory guidance and counseling, oral hygiene counseling, and referral to a dentist, but 18 states do not have a separate periodicity schedule. According to this study, those states with a separate periodicity schedule adhered more closely to the recommendations than those without. Despite best practice recommendations, only 16 states required referral to a dentist by the time a child is aged 1 year (**Table 2**).[40]

In 2013, the Center for Medicare and Medicaid Services developed a set of strategies to promote oral health for young children, including the following:

1. Improving state Medicaid program performance through policy changes such as aligning the dental periodicity schedule to clinical recommendations, reimbursing

Table 2
States with and without established timelines for dental referral under Early and Periodic Screening, Diagnosis, and Treatment

Timeline	State
Referral to a dentist by age 1	California, Colorado[a], Georgia, Idaho, Iowa, Massachusetts, Michigan[a], Missouri[a], Montana[a], New York[a], Pennsylvania, Rhode Island, Texas, Utah, Vermont, West Virginia
Referral to a dentist by age 2	Connecticut[a], Illinois, Indiana, Kentucky, Maryland[a], Nevada, Oklahoma, South Carolina[a]
Referral to a dentist by age 3	Alabama, Alaska[a], Arizona, Arkansas[a], D.C., Florida[a], Hawaii[a], Maine, Minnesota, Mississippi, Nebraska, New Jersey, New Mexico[a], North Carolina, Ohio[a], Tennessee[a], Virginia, Washington[a], Wisconsin, Wyoming
No established referral timeline	Delaware, Kansas, Louisiana, New Hampshire[a], North Dakota, Oregon, South Dakota[a]

[a] States with no separate periodicity schedule.

medical providers for preventive oral health services, incentivizing dental providers through new payment models, and addressing data collection challenges;
2. Maximizing provider participation by removing administrative burdens and helping general dentists feel more comfortable treating young children;
3. Addressing missed appointments;
4. Partnering with oral heath stakeholders.[39]

Although Medicaid covers the cost of infant oral examination and fluoride varnish application by dental professionals, variation in reimbursement rates and coding exists among states. Many states also now offer reimbursement to PCPs for fluoride varnish application for moderate- to high-risk caries patients. A small percentage pays for oral evaluation for a patient under 3 years of age and counseling with the primary caregiver as well.[42]

In the private insurance market, dental plans cover dental services provided by dental professionals. IOH examination and application of fluoride varnish are typically covered under preventive services. Based on a recent recommendation by the US Public Health Service Preventive Services Task Force, most private/commercial payers must now pay for application of topical fluoride varnish by a physician or other qualified health care professional (CPT 99188) under the health or medical plans for children up to age 6 years. This code was developed because medical health plans typically do not recognize dental service codes (D codes).[42,43]

The Affordable Care Act did little to enhance the penetration of IOH because of the legal decision to make pediatric oral health care a mandated marketplace offering rather than a mandated covered service. Consequently, it is unlikely that IOH will gain traction in the private sector without directive legislation. With consideration of block grants to states for Medicaid in this current fiscal and political environment, IOH may be at risk within Medicaid because states will likely have the option to determine which services they will offer. EPSDT may fall to a state-preferred set of services.

In an optimistic view, IOH may benefit from the movement by public funding sources to pay for performance (P4P), episodes of care, and a desire to achieve cost reductions and provide better patient experiences. As an example, a state might reward PCPs or dentists for IOH and application of fluoride varnish at regular intervals to prevent ECC and offer a capstone incentive payment to the respective provider at the end of a year of IOH visits for keeping a child out of the hospital, free of pain, and disease free. In an alternative model, for an infant with ECC but not experiencing discomfort, the P4P model may involve application of SDF with a similar set of goals. The cost of this type of approach is minor compared with the cost of general anesthesia,[5] and states may choose to incentivize IOH in a block granting scenario. In still a third scenario, public funding sources might support bundling of services for IOH with PCPs, general dentists, and pediatric dentists to support the spectrum of need that might be identified in a population from simple prevention through treatment. The lack of dental referral sources for PCPs is cited as an obstacle to its implementation.[21]

SUMMARY

Community water fluoridation may be the most recent significant preventive dental public health measure in the United States and it took decades to reach most American children. IOH may be the next best opportunity to reach children and families in an attempt to eradicate ECC. Like fluoridation, IOH reaches across all socioeconomic strata, can be implemented by medical and dental systems, and is relatively low cost, compared with the alternative of treatment of dental caries in very young children. Unlike community water fluoridation, IOH offers a value-added aspect of improved health literacy and extension of its benefits beyond the individual child with changed oral health behavior in families. It remains to be seen whether IOH will gain traction in the health community and realize its tremendous potential.

REFERENCES

1. American Academy of Pediatric Dentistry. Guideline on perinatal and infant oral health care. Pediatr Dent 2016;38:150–4.
2. American Dental Association. Mouth healthy kids. First dental visit. Available at: http://www.mouthhealthykids.org/en. Accessed March 13, 2017.
3. American Academy of Pediatrics, Section on Pediatric Dentistry and Oral health. A policy statement: preventive intervention for pediatricians. Pediatrics 2008; 122(6):1387–94.
4. Nowak AJ, Casamassimo PS. The dental home. J Am Dent Assoc 2002;133(1): 93–8.
5. Bruen BK, Steinmetz E, Bysshe T, et al. Potentially preventable dental care in operating rooms for children enrolled in Medicaid. J Am Dent Assoc 2016;147: 702–8.
6. American Academy of Pediatric Dentistry. Guideline on caries-risk assessment and management for infants, children, and adolescents. Pediatr Dent 2016; 38(6):142–9.
7. Takahashi N, Nyvad B. The role of bacteria in the caries process: ecological perspectives. J Dent Res 2011;90(3):294–303.
8. Tanzer JM, Livingston J, Thompson AM. The microbiology of primary dental caries in humans. J Dent Educ 2001;65(10):1028–37.
9. Gross EL, Beall CJ, Kutsch SR, et al. Beyond Streptococcus mutans: dental caries onset linked to multiple species by 16S rRNA community analysis. PLoS One 2012;7(10):e47722.
10. Berkowitz RJ. Mutans streptococci: acquisition and transmission. Pediatr Dent 2006;28(2):106–9.
11. Sheiham A, James WPT. Diet and dental caries: the pivotal role of free sugars reemphasized. J Dent Res 2015;94(10):1341–7.

12. Tinanoff N, Palmer CA. Dietary determinants of dental caries and dietary recommendations for preschool children. J Public Health Dent 2000;60(3):197–206.

13. Kay EJ, Vascott D, Hocking A, et al. Motivational interviewing in general dental practice: a review of the evidence. Br Dent J 2016;221(12):785–91.

14. Casamassimo PS, Thikkurissy S, Edelstein BL, et al. Beyond the DMFT: the human and economic cost of early childhood caries. J Am Dent Assoc 2009; 140(6):650–7.

16. U.S. Food and Drug Administration. FDA drug safety communication: FDA approves label changes for use of general anesthetic and sedation drugs in young children. Available at: https://www.fda.gov/Drugs/DrugSafety/ucm554634.htm. Accessed May 3, 2017.

16. Wright JT, Cutter GR, Dasanyake AP, et al. Effect of conventional dental restorative treatment on bacteria in saliva. Community Dent Oral Epidemiol 1992;20: 138–43.

17. Gregory RL, El-Rahman AMA, Avery DR. Effect of restorative treatment on mutans streptococci and IgA antibodies. Pediatr Dent 1998;20:273–7.

18. Palmer EA, Nielsen T, Peirano P, et al. Children with severe early childhood caries: pilot study examining Mutans streptococci genotypic strains after full-mouth caries restorative therapy. Pediatr Dent 2012;34(2):e1–10.

19. Belamarich PF, Gandica R, Stein REK, et al. Drowning in a sea of advice: pediatricians and American Academy of Pediatrics Policy Statements. Pediatrics 2006; 118:e964–78.

20. Dooley D, Moultrie NM, Heckman B, et al. Oral health prevention and toddler well-child care: routine integration in a safety net system. Pediatrics 2016;137(1): e20143532.

21. Lewis CW, Grossman DC, Domoto PK, et al. The role of the pediatrician in the oral health of children. Pediatrics 2000;106:e84.

22. Garg S, Rubin T, Jasek J, et al. How willing are dentists to treat young children?: a survey of dentists affiliated with Medicaid managed care in New York City, 2010. J Am Dent Assoc 2013;144(4):416–25.

23. Coe JM, Razdan S, Best AM, et al. Pediatric dentists' perspective of general dentists' role in treating children aged 0-3 years. Gen Dent 2017;65(2):e1–6.

24. Bubna S, Perez-Spiess S, Cernigliaro J, et al. Infant oral health care: beliefs and practices of American Academy of Pediatric Dentistry members. Pediatr Dent 2012;34(3):203–9.

25. Santos CL, Douglass JM. Practices and opinions of pediatric and general dentists in Connecticut regarding the age 1 dental visit and dental care for children younger than 3 years old. Pediatr Dent 2008;30(4):348–51.

26. Brickhouse TH, Unkel JH, Kancitis I, et al. Infant oral health care: a survey of general dentists, pediatric dentists, and pediatricians in Virginia. Pediatr Dent 2008; 30(2):147–53.

27. Nowak AJ, Casamassimo PS, Scott J, et al. Do early dental visits reduce treatment and treatment costs for children? Pediatr Dent 2014;36:489–93.

28. Kolstad C, Zavras A, Yoon RK. Cost-benefit analysis of the age one dental visit for the privately insured. Pediatr Dent 2015;37(4):376–80.

29. Savage MF, Lee JY, Kotch JB, et al. Early preventive dental visits: effects on subsequent utilization and costs. Pediatrics 2004;114:e418–23.

30. Blackburn J, Morrisey MA, Sen B. Outcomes associated with early preventive dental care among Medicaid-enrolled children in Alabama. JAMA Pediatr 2017; 171(4):335–41.

31. Achembong LN, Kranz AM, Rozier RG. Office-based preventive dental program and statewide trends in dental caries. Pediatrics 2014;133(4):e827–34.

32. Beil H, Rozier RG, Preisser JS, et al. Effect of early preventive dental visits on subsequent dental treatment and expenditures. Med Care 2012;50(9):749–56.

33. From the first tooth. Metrics, 2016. Available at: http://www.fromthefirsttooth.org/wp-content/uploads/2016/01/FTFT-Metrics.pdf. Accessed April 7, 2017.

34. From the first tooth website. Available at: http://www.fromthefirsttooth.org/. Accessed May 3, 2017.

35. The Pew center on the states. Washington's ABCD program: improving dental care for Medicaid-insured children. 2010. Available at: http://www.pewtrusts.org/~/media/legacy/uploadedfiles/pcs_assets/2010/abcdbriefwebpdf.pdf. Accessed April 7, 2017.

36. Braun PA, Cusick A. Collaboration between medical providers and dental hygienists in pediatric health care. J Evid Based Dent Pract 2016;16(Suppl):59–67.

37. Crystal YO, Niederman R. Silver diamine fluoride treatment considerations in children's caries management. Pediatr Dent 2016;38(7):466–71.

38. AAPD Council on Clinical Affairs. Policy on interim therapeutic restorations (ITR). Reference Manual 2016-2017. Pediatr Dent 2016;38(6):50–1.

39. Keep kids smiling: promoting oral health through the Medicaid benefit for children and adolescents. 2013. Available at: https://www.medicaid.gov/medicaid/benefits/downloads/keep-kids-smiling.pdf. Accessed April 27, 2017.

40. Center on budget and policy priorities: policy basics: introduction to Medicaid. Available at: http://www.cbpp.org/research/health/policy-basics-introduction-to-medicaid. Accessed April 22, 2017.

41. Hom JM, Lee JY, Silverman J, et al. State Medicaid early and periodic screening, diagnosis, and treatment guidelines: adherence to professionally recommended best oral health practices. J Am Dent Assoc 2013;144(3):297–305.

42. American Academy of Pediatrics. Oral health coding fact sheet for primary care physicians. 2016. Available at: https://www.aap.org/en-us/Documents/coding_factsheet_oral_health.pdf. Accessed April 27, 2017.

43. American Academy of Pediatrics. State Medicaid payment for caries prevention services by non-dental professionals. 2013. Available at: http://www2.aap.org/oralhealth/docs/OHReimbursementChart.pdf. Accessed April 27, 2017.

44. Washington Dental Service Foundation. Access to baby & child dentistry. Available at: http://abcd-dental.org/. Accessed May 3, 2017.

Dental Care for Geriatric and Special Needs Populations

Elisa M. Chávez, DDS[a],[*], Lynne M. Wong, DDS[a], Paul Subar, DDS, EdD[b],[c],
Douglas A. Young, DDS, EdD, MBA, MS[a], Allen Wong, DDS, EdD, DABSCD[d]

KEYWORDS

- Aging • Special needs • Dentistry • Oral health • Chronic disease • CAMBRA

KEY POINTS

- There are diverse health needs among older adults and adults with developmental disabilities.
- Complex health needs require an interprofessional effort.
- Oral health care can and should be provided for people with varying functional abilities and across the life span.
- Because many systemic diseases have significant direct and indirect impacts on oral health, oral health care must be an integral component of chronic disease management.

INTRODUCTION

Changing demographics, advances in medicine, and increased longevity have brought new opportunities and challenges in oral health care. Adults are retaining more of their teeth as they age, yet their oral health may be at risk or compromised due to the sequelae of acute and chronic diseases and sometimes the aging process itself.[1] The problems are compounded for populations lacking resources for oral health care. Ironically, as subsequent generations have benefited from improved oral health care and public measures to improve oral health, many are left without resources to maintain their oral health after retirement.[2] An estimated 19% of adults older than 65 have untreated dental caries, with much higher rates in Asian, Hispanic, and Black seniors ranging from 27% to 41%, respectively (2011–2012).[3] Further, if their functional status is altered by diseases, conditions, or events, they can become

Disclosures: The authors have nothing to disclose.
[a] Department of Diagnostic Sciences, University of the Pacific, Arthur A. Dugoni School of Dentistry, 155 5th Street, San Francisco, CA 94103, USA; [b] Special Care Clinic, Hospital Dentistry Program, Arthur A. Dugoni School of Dentistry, 155 5th Street, San Francisco, CA 94103, USA; [c] Department of Family and Community Medicine, UCSF School of Medicine, San Francisco, CA, USA; [d] AEGD Program, Hospital Dentistry Program, University of the Pacific, Arthur A. Dugoni School of Dentistry, 155 5th Street, San Francisco, CA 94103, USA
* Corresponding author.
E-mail address: echavez@pacific.edu

Dent Clin N Am 62 (2018) 245–267
https://doi.org/10.1016/j.cden.2017.11.005
0011-8532/18/© 2018 Elsevier Inc. All rights reserved.

more vulnerable to oral diseases. Certain populations have chronically had limited re-sources for dental care or limited understanding of its importance.[1] Aging adults with special needs have often lived their lifetime with disparities in, and risks to, their oral health.[4] Although these issues are complex, we review approaches to oral health care that consider the health and functional status of each individual and carefully assess risk so that providers feel confident to plan and provide appropriate, safe care to diverse populations at any stage of life.[5]

APPROPRIATE TREATMENT PLANNING

There are 2 treatment-planning schemas that are especially useful for older adults. One is OSCAR: "The Five-Point Geriatric Dental Assessment."[6] The acronym guides the practitioner to consider 5 key areas in the oral health plan and management: Oral, Systemic, Capability, Autonomy, Reality. Although every patient requires a thorough assessment of the oral cavity (oral) and health history (systemic) to provide safe and appropriate treatment, for adults with complex needs, considering the patient's ability for self-care (capability) and to consent to care (autonomy) are crucial to planning appropriate treatment. Although most patients must consider their finances, these patients may have additional considerations, such as life expectancy and palliative or end-of-life care (reality).[6] In addition, patient and surrogate decision makers' perceptions around their need for dental care can play a role in the acceptance or refusal of dental treatment. Many view oral health care as optional or believe that oral health is bound to decline with aging,[7] so practitioners must carefully discuss with their patients the causes of oral diseases and reinforce that tooth loss is not an inevitable nor a part of normal aging.[8]

The Seattle Care Pathway (SCP) also helps practitioners evaluate their patients' functional status and then consider the resultant risks to their oral health.[5] Based on functional status designation (none, pre, low, medium, or high dependency) SCP offers recommendations for the type of prevention and treatment that is appropriate at each stage. Additionally, it guides practitioners to engage with other health care providers to gather and give information that will improve outcomes as dependency increases. An overview is provided in **Table 1**. Importantly, SCP allows practitioners to consider that well elders, those who are not dependent and with few oral health risks as a result of systemic disease, can benefit from and tolerate routine oral health care regardless of their age.[5]

CARIES MANAGEMENT BY RISK ASSESSMENT AND MINIMALLY INVASIVE DENTISTRY

Dental caries is a complex, multifactorial disease that is usually chronic and progressive in nature. The expression of the disease on the teeth (caries lesions) is determined by balance or imbalance between protective biological factors (such as salivary flow, buffering capacity, healthy biofilm, fluoride, genetics, and host immunity) and pathogenic factors that put teeth at increased risk (such as frequent exposure to dietary carbohydrates, poor oral hygiene, cariogenic biofilm, and salivary dysfunction resulting in a low salivary pH and/or buffering capacity).[9,10] Caries management by risk assessment (CAMBRA) is an evidence-based philosophy that uses the patient's unique caries risk profile to prevent, reverse, and, when necessary, repair damage to teeth using tooth preserving, minimally invasive methodologies.[11] There is consensus internationally that the evidence clearly supports less invasive carious lesion management compared with traditional methods of placing restorations only.[12] This may include delaying surgical restoration and using more conservative caries removal techniques.[12] Partial caries removal[13] in a selective manner is

Table 1
Seattle Care Pathway (SCP) overview

Implementation	No Dependency: They Are the Most Fit in Their Age Group	Predependency: the Disease(s) Is Controlled but with Potential to Impact Oral Health	Low Dependency: the Systemic Disease(s) Is Impacting Oral Health but No Obvious Dependence	Medium Dependency: the Systemic Disease Is Impacting Oral Health, They Require Some Support to Access Care and Maintain Oral Health	High Dependency: the Systemic Disease Impacts Oral Health and Prevents Oral Health Care
Assessment of risks to oral health	Recall and risk assessment to standard of care	Specific risks to oral health from the disease(s) and its management and reevaluation of the current preventive plan	Identify cause of dependency and associated risk(s), increased recall, prepare for change in preventive plan	Recognition that increased dependency increases risk, include other providers, that is, interdisciplinary team (IDT) to address risks, reassess prevention plan	Identify barriers to care and monitor, potential for abuse
Prevention plan	Patient performs routine homecare	Possible implementation of prescription (Rx) preventives and specific oral hygiene (OH) instruction and (OH) plan	Identify cause of risk, modify plan as needed, consider role of polypharmacy, Rx preventives, OH plan	Increased involvement of the IDT, review polypharmacy for risks, Rx and professionally applied preventives, daily OH plan	Rx and professionally applied preventive, risk specific daily OH
Treatment goals	Routine standard of care for dental need	Create a long-term plan for restorative and maintenance care	Restore and maintain function	Increased minimally invasive care and focus on preservation; however, viability of more complex care should be considered	Focus is palliative care, maintenance of dignity and comfort
Communication	Direct patient education	Discuss potential oral complications related disease(s) or its management directly with the patient	Identify others who can participate in prevention with the patient	IDT focus on ensuring support for a daily care plan provided by the patient or caregiver as needed	All providers and caregivers involved to ensure well-being of the patient

Based on levels of dependency, SCP recommends risk assessments needed, appropriate preventive measures, and treatment considerations and a guide to what information should be provided to whom at each stage of dependency.
Data from Pretty IA, Ellwood RP, Lo E, et al. The Seattle care pathway for securing oral health in older patients. Gerodontology 2014;31(s1):77–87.

preferred and sometimes no caries removal may be indicated.[12] This can be especially helpful in frail populations or those not able to tolerate or cooperate for extensive dental treatment.[5]

CLINICAL EXAMINATION AND CARIES RISK ASSESSMENT

Diagnosis and management of disease starts with a careful patient interview and hard
tissue examination, which must be done before completing a caries risk assessment
(CRA). The CRA process will determine the chance of future caries activity, but it also
determines the pathogenic risk factors that need to be treated to manage the disease.
The most powerful predictor of future caries lesion development is past caries experience.[14] The presence of any new or progressing caries lesions are considered high
caries risk. However, just knowing someone is high risk does not give you helpful information on preventing the next caries lesion. For this we need to identify and reduce
the pathogenic risk factors. The 3 obvious caries risk factors are (1) acidogenic biofilm
behavior, (2) absence of saliva, and (3) destructive lifestyle habits (eg, due to poor diet,
drug use, dependence on others). In contrast to medicine, treating risk factors is a
fairly new approach in managing caries disease in which the current economic model
rewards the traditional "drill and fill" restorative approach and does little to treat and
prevent the underlying disease.[15] Some specific risks factors exist for special needs,
medically compromised, and older patients. Some patients may have poor oral hygiene as a result of some physical or cognitive impairment. Some patients may require
special diets, such as mechanical soft, puree, or thickened liquids because of certain
health conditions. This could be a temporary or permanent situation, but in either case
places the patient at risk for caries activity because of the difficulty of removing such
foods from the tooth surfaces. Importantly, those who are tube fed are still at risk for
caries if they have teeth and can still benefit from CRA and require a daily oral care
plan.[16]

Often special needs, medically compromised, and older patients are considered
extreme caries risk, which is by definition a high-risk patient who also has diminished
salivary flow by observation or measurement.[10] This can result in multiple advanced
caries lesions (rampant decay), especially on root surfaces. After a CRA is properly
performed, risk-based treatment options, often including products, are recommended
to reduce the patients' pathogenic risk factors.[17]

Using the principles of CAMBRA to control of the disease during the restorative
phase is critical. To restore teeth without addressing the cause will not stop new lesions
in the future.[15] In addition to chemical CAMBRA interventions, which patients use on
their own, patients with multiple advanced lesions often require additional materials
or techniques, such as silver diamine fluoride and conventional glass ionomer cement
(as described in Jeremy A. Horst and colleagues' article, "Fluorides and Other
Preventive Strategies for Tooth Decay," in this issue), used independently or in combination to chemically treat caries lesions by remineralization. Such efforts are appropriate for patients less able to tolerate traditional restorative techniques as well.[15]

COMMON COMORBIDITIES AND IMPLICATIONS FOR CARE

OSCAR, SCP, and CAMBRA provide practitioners valuable guidance in managing
populations that are widely heterogeneous and complex.[5,6,15] National vital statistics
for 2014 show the top 5 causes of death among those older than 65 were cardiovascular disease, cancer, chronic lower respiratory diseases (chronic obstructive pulmonary disease [COPD]), cerebrovascular disease, and Alzheimer disease (AD).[18]
Diabetes mellitus (DM), types 1 and 2, and renal and liver diseases are also significant

causes of illness and death among older adults.[18] We review the most common causes and the associated considerations for oral health and oral health care. All of these diseases can be debilitating in advanced stages and present significant risks to oral health and complications in the provision of effective and safe oral health care.[8] **Table 2** frames DM and renal and liver diseases within the context of the SCP to demonstrate increasing disability along with concomitant challenges to oral health care needs and treatment considerations.[5,8,19–26] It should be noted that these are *examples* of a continuum of declining function. The examples are not intended as definitive assignment of a disease stage to a dependency status. Clinicians must use their clinical judgment, in consultation with other health providers to determine individual patient functional status and needs as they apply the principles of SCP.[5]

Older adults and those with special needs also contend with several chronic impairments, such as hearing and vision impairments, altered chemosensory function, orthopedic impairments, and oral motor function problems.[24,27] **Table 3** highlights the oral health risks and considerations in the provision of care for individuals with these impairments, as well as for those with diminished salivary flow, which also is common among older adults as a result of disease or medication use.[5,28] Each of these impairments compound the risks to oral health for people with systemic diseases.[27] And, many of the risk factors for systemic diseases, for example, excess sugar intake, obesity, poor diet, substance dependence, and socioeconomic determinants of health, also carry risk for poor oral health.[29] By understanding the causes of most commonly occurring comorbidities and conditions in these populations and their implications for oral health, we can provide safe, efficient, and appropriate care at every level of function and age.

CARDIOVASCULAR DISEASE

Cardiovascular disease has many risk factors, including congenital, genetic, cholesterol, diet, exercise, smoking, gender, race, and stress. Infective endocarditis, hypertension, ischemic heart disease, arrhythmias, and heart failure are all forms of heart disease.[19] Atherosclerosis or thickening of the vascular vessels with plaque can create additional hemodynamic pressures and is detected as hypertension. Hypertension is a common problem in older adults, with a prevalence of 60% to 80%, and it is anticipated to increase.[30] Atherosclerotic cardiovascular disease risk factors are prevalent in adults with congenital heart disease as well.[30] Patients with hypertension are usually medication controlled along with lifestyle adjustments, including diet, exercise, and stress reduction. Common medications for hypertension include diuretics, beta-blockers, angiotensin-converting enzyme (ACE) inhibitors/angiotensin receptor blockers, aldosterone antagonists, and blood thinners. Hypertension can lead to serious symptoms, including angina (lack of oxygen to the heart) and myocardial infarction. Uncontrolled hypertension can lead to stress in other organ systems and compromise their function. Increased blood pressure can damage the blood vessels, including rupture (aneurysm) or blockage in major organs such as the brain (stroke) and the heart (heart attacks).[30]

Implications for Oral Health and Treatment

Medications that treat cardiovascular disease often reduce salivary flow or cause xerostomia, resulting in discomfort, candidal infection, halitosis, and an increased risk for caries and soft tissue trauma.[31] Some medications may cause an overgrowth of gingival tissues (calcium channel blockers), altered taste (ACE inhibitors) or risk for bleeding gingiva or excessive postoperative bleeding (anticoagulants). Drugs

Table 2
Declining functional status as a result of diabetes mellitus, renal and liver diseases, and implications for oral health care

Disease	Impact on the Oral Cavity	Considerations in Patient Care	Disease Progression and Severity in the Framework of the Seattle Pathway[a]
Diabetes mellitus (type1, type 2)	Candida Dysphagia Taste disorders Burning mouth Poor wound healing increased risk of infection Periodontal disease caries Diminished salivary flow Consider: Frequent dental evaluations Caries risk assessment Avoid dry or acidic foods Rx oral antibacterial Fluoride Xylitol Calcium/phosphate and pH neutralizing products	Confirm patient has followed usual medication (especially insulin)/meal routine before appointments. Consult patient's physician if an altered regimen is needed. Consider glucose check in office. Oral infections can make glucose management problematic. Blood glucose can rise with the administration of local anesthetics with epinephrine. For extensive surgery, consider a course of antibiotics for patients with poor control. Signs of Hyperglycemia (Blood glucose higher than 200): Frequent urination Extreme thirst Dry skin Hunger Blurred vision Drowsiness Nausea	Predependency: disease is controlled but with potential to impact oral health: prescription preventives and formal oral care plan, patient informed of risks to oral health. Low dependency: systemic disease is impacting oral health: identify risk factors for oral diseases, including polypharmacy; prescription preventives and formal oral care plan. Target for HbA1C: which measures long-term control is typically 7%; however, the target may be higher for older and frail adults. Medium dependency: systemic disease is impacting oral health and help is needed to access or maintain oral health: include interdisciplinary team in prevention as appropriate, identify risk factors for oral diseases, including polypharmacy; prescription preventives and formal oral care plan.

Ketoacidosis is life-threatening and needs immediate medical treatment.

Symptoms include

Shortness of breath

Breath that smells fruity

Nausea and vomiting

Very dry mouth

Signs of hypoglycemia (blood glucose <70):

Mild:

Hunger

Weakness

Tachycardia

Pallor

Sweating

Paresthesia

Moderate:

Incoherence

Uncooperative

Belligerence

Lack of judgment

Poor orientation

Severe:

Loss of consciousness

Tonic/clonic movements

Hypotension

Hypothermia

Rapid, thread pulse[2]

Have a source of glucose available and be prepared to initiate an emergency response for patients with severe hypoglycemia.

The uncontrolled patient has fasting glucose <70 or >200.

Neuropathies, retinopathies, and nephropathy begin to impact functional status.

High dependency: systemic disease is preventing the receipt of oral health care: assess unique barriers to oral care, aggressive prevention, include interdisciplinary team in prevention and palliative care as appropriate, identify risk factors for oral diseases, including polypharmacy prescription preventives and formal oral care plan.

Patients with recent history of myocardial infarction, cerebrovascular accident, renal disease, congestive heart failure, unstable angina, or blood pressure >180/110 should only have appropriate emergency and palliative dental services offered until medical condition(s) have stabilized and under the guidance of physician.

(continued on next page)

Table 2
(continued)

Disease	Impact on the Oral Cavity	Considerations in Patient Care	Disease Progression and Severity in the Framework of the Seattle Pathway[a]
Renal diseases End-stage renal disease (ESRD) occurs most commonly in patients with both diabetes mellitus and hypertension Other causes of ESRD include chronic glomerulonephritis Polycystic kidney disease Systemic lupus erythematosus, kidney neoplasms.[3]	Xerostomia; pigmented oral mucosa; dysgeusia; candida; petechiae; uremic stomatitis; lichen planus; hairy tongue; increased risk of pyogenic granulomas Radiolucent jaw lesions (hyperparathyroidism) Consider: Frequent dental evaluations Caries risk assessment Avoid dry or acidic foods Rx oral antibacterial Fluoride Xylitol Calcium/phosphate and pH neutralizing products	Identify placement of shunt and avoid when taking blood pressure. Possibly diminished platelet count and function. Patient fatigue and temporary coagulation disturbance on dialysis days, avoid routine care on the day of hemodialysis treatment. Small risk of infection at the catheter. Corticosteroid supplementation of immunosuppressed patient posttransplantation. Consult regarding any question of premedication. Use proper surgical technique. Avoid trauma to soft tissues. Place hemostatic packing material into extraction sites with appropriate suture placement. Aggressive management of orofacial infections. Dose alterations for drugs metabolized by the kidney, such as amoxicillin, penicillin, cephalosporin. GFR <10 mL/min 1 dose every 24 h. 10–50 mL/min 1 dose every 8–12 h. >50 mL/min 1 dose every 8 h.	Predependency: disease is controlled but with potential to impact oral health: prescription preventives and formal oral care plan, patient informed of risks to oral health. Renal insufficiency. Low dependency: systemic disease is impacting oral health: identify risk factors for oral diseases including polypharmacy; prescription preventives and formal oral care plan. Stage 1 chronic kidney disease (CKD) Decrease of glomerular filtration rate (GFR) 10%. Asymptomatic, minimal clinical significance. Hypertension, mild fluid retention. Stage 2 (CKD) Decrease of GFR 20%–40%. Accumulation of nitrogen compounds. Increase of blood urea nitrogen. Metabolic acidosis. Patient hyperventilation. Mild anemia. Slightly impaired platelet function. Slightly impaired coagulation factors. Mild white blood cell destruction. Nausea and vomiting. Fatigue.

Medium dependency: systemic disease is impacting oral health and help is needed to access or maintain oral health: include interdisciplinary team in prevention as appropriate, identify risk factors for oral diseases including polypharmacy; prescription preventives and formal oral care plan.

Stage 3a (CKD)/ESRD

Decrease of GFF 50%.

All of the above, including

Early congestive heart failure.

Fluid retention in extremities.

Dialysis.

High dependency: systemic disease is preventing the receipt of oral health care: assess unique barriers to oral care, aggressive prevention, include interdisciplinary team in prevention and palliative care as appropriate, identify risk factors for oral diseases including polypharmacy prescription preventives and formal oral care plan.

Stage 3b (CKD)/ESRD:

Decrease of GFR 60%–70%.

Congestive heart failure.

Dialysis.

Stage 4 ESRD:

Decrease of GFR 80%.

Severe effect on organ systems.

Stage 5 kidney failure:

Decrease of GFR >90%.

Severe congestive heart failure.

Transplant.

(continued on next page)

Table 2
(continued)

Disease	Impact on the Oral Cavity	Considerations in Patient Care	Disease Progression and Severity in the Framework of the Seattle Pathway[a]
Liver diseases Hepatitis Substance related Neoplasm Poisoning Medication overdose	Hyposalivation Xerostomia Gastric reflux Erosion Poor wound healing prolonged bleeding periodontitis Increased oral infections Consider: Frequent dental evaluations Caries risk assessment Avoid dry or acidic foods Rx oral antibacterial Fluoride Xylitol Calcium/phosphate and pH neutralizing products	Platelets and INR (international normalized ratio) need to be in a therapeutic range (within 48 h of the procedure) to facilitate clotting. Review of the patient's coagulation status should be requested, and necessary precautions made (eg, blood products and/or antibiotics) before a procedure. Consider hospital dentistry if unprepared to manage severe bleeding. Symptoms of cirrhosis can include: Fluid retention Easily bruised Jaundice Development of insulin-resistant diabetes Problems with concentration and memory. Early symptoms of liver failure: Loss of appetite, nausea, fatigue, diarrhea. Symptoms of acute liver failure: Confusion, disorientation, sleepiness, coma, and death.	Predependency: disease is controlled but with potential to impact oral health: prescription preventives and formal oral care plan, patient informed of risks to oral health. Fibrosis. Low dependency: systemic disease is impacting oral health: identify risk factors for oral diseases including polypharmacy; prescription preventives and formal oral care plan. Cirrhosis. Medium dependency: systemic disease is impacting oral health and help is needed to access or maintain oral health: include interdisciplinary team in prevention as appropriate, identify risk factors for oral diseases including polypharmacy; prescription preventives and formal oral care plan. Advanced cirrhosis.

Liver function tests: aspartate transaminase, alanine transaminase (liver transaminases). If tests are 4 times greater than normal, do not use drugs metabolized by or toxic to the liver, such as lidocaine, acetaminophen, codeine, lorazepam, ketoconazole.

High dependency: systemic disease is preventing the receipt of oral health care: assess unique barriers to oral care, aggressive prevention, include interdisciplinary team in prevention and palliative care as appropriate, identify risk factors for oral diseases including polypharmacy; prescription preventives and formal oral care plan.
Liver failure and/or transplant.

[a] These are examples of a continuum of declining function and the impact on oral health and the provision of care. Clinicians must use clinical judgment, in consultation with other health providers to determine individual patient status and needs as they apply the principles of SCP.
Data from Refs.[5,8,19–26]

Table 3
Common chronic conditions in older adults that can impact oral health

Condition	Oral Health Concerns	Risk Factor for	Modifications/Considerations
Xerostomia Salivary gland hypofunction Disease or medication related	Impaired mastication, speaking, and swallowing; complaint of taste disorders, sore throat, or burning sensation; salivary gland retention or infection	Periodontal disease; dental caries/root caries; dental erosion; candidiasis; poor retention of removable prosthodontics; soft tissue trauma	Frequent dental and oral evaluations; diet low in sugar and avoid dry or acidic foods; avoid caffeine-containing or alcoholic beverages Use of oral antibacterial, fluoride, xylitol, calcium/phosphate, and pH neutralizing products as needed Assistance from caregivers with oral hygiene as needed; increased use of professionally applied products Pain and infection management; prevention of disease complication Referral to other health care provider
Hearing impairment Age and/or disease related	Compromised communication between patient and caregiver, resulting in poor home care, inadequate postoperative care, and fear and anxiety in clinic setting	Poor oral hygiene; periodontal disease; dental caries; postoperative complications	Clinician should face patient directly when speaking; enunciate words clearly and speak slowly; discussions in a quiet setting; written instructions; do not speak as if to a child Referral to other health care provider
Visual impairment Age and/or disease related	Decreased ability to evaluate own oral hygiene or detect oral problems by sight Could compromise compliance Possibly related to other diseases that also impact oral health: diabetes, Sjogren syndrome	Poor oral hygiene; periodontal disease; dental caries; postoperative complications	Read forms to patient, patient/education material in larger and bold print, remove barriers to help with ambulation and assist patient in the dental office Frequent dental and oral evaluations Assistance from caregivers with oral hygiene as needed; increased use of professionally applied products Referral to other health care provider

Orthopedic impairment Advanced age and/or disease related	Impeded mobility and dexterity required for daily oral hygiene and regular dental visit; Chronic or high-dose nonsteroidal anti-inflammatory drug use could increase risk of bleeding during certain procedures; Temporomandibular joint can also be impacted	Poor oral hygiene; periodontal disease; dental caries	Frequent dental and oral evaluations; larger toothbrush handles, electric toothbrush, interproximal cleaning devices, oral irrigation devices; Use of oral antibacterial, fluoride, xylitol, calcium/phosphate, and pH neutralizing products as needed; Assistance from caregivers with oral hygiene as needed; increased use of professionally applied products; Pain and infection management; consideration of prevention of disease complication; Referral to other health care provider
Oral motor disturbance Age and/or disease related	Affect food preferences, perceived ease of chewing, taste, and texture acceptability; increased risk of dysphagia; increased risk of aspiration pneumonia	Poor oral hygiene, periodontal disease; dental caries/root caries	Frequent dental and oral evaluations; maintaining an intact dentition and chewing ability; Assistance from caregivers with oral hygiene; increased use of professional applied products, such as oral antibacterial, fluoride, xylitol, calcium/phosphate, and pH neutralizing products as needed; Pain and infection management; consideration of prevention of disease complication; Referral to other health care provider
Taste and smell dysfunction Age and/or disease related	Altered nutritional intake, indifferent to eating; Choosing more pleasing food textures or flavors; Eating for only social or health reasons	Poor oral hygiene, periodontal disease; dental caries/root caries	Frequent dental and oral evaluations; make food more appealing: presentation, temperature, texture; Assistance from caregivers with oral hygiene; increased use of professionally applied products, such as oral antibacterial, fluoride, xylitol, calcium/phosphate, and pH neutralizing products as needed; Pain and infection management; consideration of prevention of disease complication; Referral to other health care provider

Data from Refs.[25,27,28]

prescribed to prevent blood clots may require recent bloodwork to confirm a low risk of excessive bleeding (eg, international normalized ratio [INR] for Coumadin [warfarin] within 48 hours of surgery) and/or close attention to surgical technique to avoid excessive bleeding when reliable laboratory tests are not available (eg, Plavix [clopidogrel] and Eliquis [apixaban]).[19] Discontinuation of anticoagulants is not typically required.

Panoramic radiographs (Panorex) have been suggested to evaluate carotid plaques at routine dental check-ups. Early detection of these plaques may help prevent premature cardiovascular disease.[32] Patients with such findings on a routine dental examination should be referred to their primary care provider for additional evaluation and follow-up.

For patients with well-controlled cardiovascular disease, routine preventive and restorative care is appropriate.[5] However, some precautions should be taken. Older adults can be prone to orthostatic hypotension, so after lengthy appointments they should be brought slowly to an upright position. They should confirm they do not feel dizzy before standing. For those patients on nonselective beta-blockers or those with angina, epinephrine-impregnated packing cords should be avoided and epinephrine at 1:100,000 solutions should be limited to 2 or fewer cartridges. Patients taking digoxin may experience arrhythmias when epinephrine is used. Because stress can induce arrhythmias and raise blood pressure, anxiolytics also may be considered.[19] Short-acting benzodiazepines should be considered for older adults because clearance may take longer, resulting in prolonged sedation and risk for adverse events, such as falls or other accidents.[33] Prophylactic antibiotics are considered only for those at highest risk of infective endocarditis and they should be encouraged to maintain optimal oral hygiene as an additional preventive measure.[19]

When cardiovascular disease is uncontrolled, options are often limited to palliative care only or removal of infectious teeth and avoidance of complex treatment that may or may not be successful. Replacement teeth may not be a high priority in these instances.[5] Elective treatment should be deferred for patients with pressures higher than 180/110.[19] In the meantime, an aggressive preventive plan should be in place that is appropriate to the patient's functional status and the risks to their oral health during that period.[5] Elective dental care can be resumed 1 month post myocardial infarction without symptoms and with appropriate precautions; however, the physician should be consulted to confirm the severity of the event and stability of the patient's condition.[19]

CANCER

Improvement in diagnosis and treatment of cancer has improved survival rates, but cancer continues to be a major cause of morbidity and mortality. Breast, lung, and prostate cancers are the most common.[34] In 2016, oral cancer was estimated to account for 2.5% of all cancers. It is more prevalent in older adults.[35] The 5-year survival rate for oropharyngeal cancers is estimated at 64%.[2,36] Current therapies for malignant conditions can produce profound effects on normal oral tissues, such as mucositis, xerostomia, and trismus. The oral mucosa and salivary system are especially susceptible to the effects of chemotherapy and radiation treatment.[37,38] Significant oral symptoms may result in interruption of cancer therapy to allow for patients to rehydrate or maintain basic nutrition.[38]

Implications for Oral Health and Treatment

Treatment for malignancies often includes a combination of chemotherapy, radiation, surgical intervention, or a combination. Although head and neck cancer and its treatment results in the most profound changes to oral health and homeostasis. Chemotherapy for non–head and neck cancers can result in significant changes, including mucositis, xerostomia, dysgeusia, and pain. These conditions can contribute to dysphagia, rampant caries, dehydration, and malnutrition. Osteoradionecrosis (ORN) is a significant complication of head and neck radiation and occurs due to damage of the fine vasculature surrounding dental structures from ionizing radiation, typically in doses more than 5500 cGy. Bone remodeling becomes impaired, and following surgery or trauma or sometimes spontaneously, the bone becomes necrotic. Depending on severity, treatment may include ostectomy/sequestrectomy or microvascular transfer.[1,37,38] Radiation to other areas of the body do not result in ORN in the orofacial region or salivary gland damage.[38]

A multidisciplinary approach is best before, during, and after cancer treatment. The multidisciplinary team includes but is not limited to oncologists, radiation oncologists, dentists, hygienists, dieticians, and social workers. The main objective for precancer treatment is to stabilize or eliminate/minimize oral disease before the initiation of cancer treatment. Comprehensive oral health care should be provided ahead of cancer therapy when possible and could include CRA, oral prophylaxis, scaling/root planning, extraction of nonrestorable teeth or those with a guarded or poor endodontic/periodontal prognosis, restorative dentistry, evaluation and adjustment of removable appliances, fabrication of custom fluoride trays, and intensive, ongoing oral hygiene instruction.[38] Intracancer treatment management focuses on palliative treatment (not including dental extractions); continuing intensive CAMBRA regimen; and frequent recall visits to manage pain, mucositis, trismus, dysgeusia, xerostomia, and fungal infections.[37,39] Routine dentistry can be resumed after cancer therapy has ended and the patient's condition has stabilized. Indicators of stability may include neutrophils returning to more than 2000/mm^3,[37] and platelet levels to a threshold of more than 60K and approaching normal low range of 150K. Restorative dentistry, reconstructive dentistry, and dental extractions can be considered when platelet number, function, and neutrophil numbers have stabilized.[37,39] However, if a tooth in the field of radiation is to be extracted, there can be a significant risk of ORN if the dose to the tooth was more than 5500 cGy.[37,39] Patients may experience a life-long risk of oral complications, such as severe xerostomia, which is a risk factor for oral diseases and a source of discomfort. The multidisciplinary team should communicate continually through the cancer treatment and beyond to provide appropriate care for patients who may continue to need their support over a lifetime.[37]

CHRONIC OBSTRUCTIVE PULMONARY DISEASES

COPD, which includes chronic bronchitis and emphysema, is the third leading cause of death in the United States.[18] Chronic bronchitis is more prevalent, affecting 9.5 million people, and emphysema affecting 3.5 million people. COPD-related deaths occur more often in men than women, but both genders have shown increased risk of death from COPD over the past 15 years.[40] Although smoking is a major factor in COPD, 20% of patients with COPD are nonsmokers.[41] Obstruction is caused by the narrowing of small airways, increased sputum production, mucus plugging, and collapse of peripheral airways. Chronic bronchitis is characterized by excessive mucus production, and a chronic cough with sputum production for a least 3 months for the past 2 years. Obstruction is present on inspiration and expiration. Emphysema is a distension of the air spaces distal to the terminal bronchioles due to destruction of alveolar septa.[41] Emphysema involves injury to alveolar epithelium. Inflammatory mediators caused by smoking induce the production of neutrophils that then release the enzyme elastase, which leads to destruction of pulmonary alveolar walls and loss of elastic recoil. Obstruction is caused by the collapse of unsupported air spaces on expiration.[41]

There is no cure for either chronic bronchitis or emphysema. Smoking cessation is the primary recommendation on diagnosis. Regular exercise, maintaining good nutrition, and aggressive treatment of respiratory infections are indicated. Patients with COPD are often on low-flow oxygen to maintain minimal oxygenation. Common medications for the patient with COPD include both inhaled and/or systemic corticosteroids, as well as antileukotrienes, bronchodilators, epinephrine, ephedrine, and B_2 agonists, both short term and long term.[19]

Implications for Oral Health and Treatment

There are several recommendations to keep in mind when managing the oral health of a patient with COPD. These include providing proper anesthesia; using pulse oximetry to monitor oxygen saturation if the patient has severe COPD; providing low-flow oxygen, 2 to 3 L/min; avoiding elective dentistry if the patient has an upper respiratory infection; avoiding a reclined chair position to ease the burden of breathing; avoiding rubber dams in the severely affected patient; avoiding nitrous/oxygen in the patient with severe COPD and use with caution in mildly affected individuals; and avoiding several drug classes, including narcotics, antihistamines, and anticholinergics, which have the potential for producing respiratory depression and/or thickened mucus.[19] Because these diseases are associated with a history of smoking, patients should have regular screenings for oral cancer.[29]

CEREBROVASCULAR

Strokes kill more than 140,000 Americans each year, accounting for 1 of 20 deaths. They are the leading cause of disability with more than half of those 65 or older having diminished mobility or other functional and cognitive impairments.[42,43] Cerebrovascular disease is a decrease or occlusion of blood flow to the brain. Atherosclerosis in the vessels can inflame or cause a decrease in blood flow, impairing the function of the brain by decreased oxygen, leading to a transient ischemic attack (TIA) or if completely blocked by a clot or an air bubble, resulting in an ischemic stroke. Hemorrhagic strokes occur when a vessel ruptures.[44]

The symptoms of cerebrovascular disease depend on the location of the affected lesion. Typical signs of a cerebrovascular attack (CVA) include altered motor or sensory function in half the body, that is, hemiplegia or hemiparesis. A person experiencing a CVA (stroke) can have a sense of disorientation. A guide for identifying a person who has had or is having a stroke is the FAST mnemonic: Face, Arms, Speech, and Time.[45] Look at the person. Have the person smile, if the face shows an asymmetric smile, it may indicate weakness in the facial muscles on one side. Have the patient close his or her eyes and raise both arms and see if one arm to drifts downward. Next, have the patient repeat a simple phrase and listen for slurred or strange speech. Last, remember that time is crucial to getting help; call 911 immediately.[19]

Implications for Oral Health and Treatment

Treatment for prevention of strokes is primarily with platelet inhibitors, such as aspirin, ticlopidine, clopidogrel, or anticoagulants such as Warfarin.[19] Laboratory work should be ordered to assess the risk of excessive bleeding during or following a procedure that may cause bleeding, such as extractions or deep scaling. A PFA-100 can be requested for patients taking aspirin therapy, and a prothrombin time (PT) (normal range is 10–12 seconds, although this can vary) and INR (normal range is 1–2, and takes into account the variation in PT results from laboratory to laboratory). These should be taken no more than 48 hours prior to surgery for those patients taking warfarin (Coumadin). Although there are no recommended treatment modifications for several drugs such as clopidogrel (Plavix) and apixaban (Eliquis), there is still the potential for complications, such as excessive bleeding and ecchymosis following procedures, and rarely neutropenia and thrombocytopenia.[19]

The general health condition of the patient and the procedure should be taken into consideration when evaluating the risk of providing treatment to a patient on anticoagulants. If the patient is having extensive oral surgery, or has multiple conditions or medications that may impair coagulation, it may be best to treat at an INR of 3.0 or less, or refer the patient to an oral surgeon and/or complete the treatment in a hospital setting if significant bleeding is anticipated.[19] The patient's physician should be consulted if altering the medication is thought to be necessary. Practitioners should use their knowledge of the patient's history as well as knowledge about their own skills in making these treatment decisions. Surgical technique to minimize trauma can minimize risk of excessive bleeding. The use of topical hemostatic agents, such as gel foam or Surgicel also should be considered. Suturing to primary closure is appropriate especially in patients who also may be cognitively or physically impaired and cannot follow postoperative instructions.[8] Carefully review postoperative instructions with the patient, or the patient's caregiver, to be sure that the caregiver does not inadvertently disrupt the clotting process after the patient has left the office.

Patients who are left with residual functional impairment as a result of a stroke may be challenged to provide their own oral hygiene, care for prostheses, or even use prostheses if they have significant oral motor dysfunction.[19,27] Treatment planning with these needs in mind is a critical step in making certain an appropriate treatment plan and home care plan are recommended.[5,8] It is important to consider that risk for another stoke is higher in the first 6 months, so elective care and definitive treatment planning should be delayed during this recovery period.[19] Patients who suffered significant functional and cognitive impairments may improve during this time, so other treatment options may become possible, and an aggressive preventive plan based on their risks[17] should be in place for patients until they can resume routine care.

DEMENTIA

AD is the most common cause of dementia and a leading cause of death in the United States.[18] The disease progressively destroys cognitive skills.[46] The causes and mechanisms of dementia are complex.[47] A broad understanding the type of dementia and the expected progression of the disease from a clinical perspective is important in management, as well as treatment planning.[5,6,8] For example, vascular dementia can occur as a sudden onset resulting from a CVA or TIA.[47] If future events can be prevented by lifestyle changes on other treatment to prevent vascular events, then the extent and severity of the patient's dementia may remain stable. Advancement can occur, but it is not a given as it is for AD and Parkinson-related dementia, which are progressive. Individuals with AD will eventually rely on others for their basic activities of daily living. There are no treatments at present that cure or reverse the course of AD. The therapies available only slow the onset of symptoms or target behavioral symptoms, but all areas of cognition will decline over time, and as the disease advances, patients may be prescribed antidepressants, antipsychotics, and anxiolytics,[46] all of which can impact oral health and the provision of dental care.[8]

Implications for Oral Health and Treatment

Ideally patients would have a dental evaluation in the predependent stages[5] of the disease when the patient is better able to follow instructions, adapt to change, and make decisions. Restorative and prosthodontic treatment should be completed as early in the disease as possible. A thorough preventive plan must be implemented and modified as the disease progresses.[5] In advanced stages, these patients will be at greater risk for caries, oral pathology, and periodontal disease due to lack of motivation and understanding, dietary restrictions, and reliance on others for oral care compounded by behavior that may prevent oral care.[5,6,8] Patients in advanced stages also may suffer orofacial trauma from falls and other accidental injury. Carefully assess whether or not the patient can follow postoperative instructions to prevent self-inflicted injury after local anesthesia and postoperative bleeding. Gathering input from other providers, caregivers, and family members before finalizing treatment plans for patients with dementia can be valuable.[5,6] This is also an opportunity to discuss the limitations of treatment due to the kind and severity of dementia as well as the behavioral or sedation interventions that may be required to complete desired or needed treatment. Treatment goals in later stages may be focused on prevention and the preservation of comfort and dignity, such as medication or rinses to relieve pain or discomfort or the use of soft relines of prostheses to relieve discomfort and/or prolong their use.[5]

SPECIAL ISSUES
Polypharmacy

Older adults and adults with special needs who also have multiple comorbid chronic conditions also will present with polypharmacy. Polypharmacy can refer to taking multiple medications at once or taking 1 or more medications incorrectly. Studies have shown the risk of adverse reactions rising dramatically with the number of medications taken. In addition to calling our attention to the number and severity of systemic diseases a patient has, there are several broad issues to consider when managing patients taking multiple prescription and over-the-counter medications.[33]

1. Some patients will have prescriptions that are needed during an emergency; that is, nitroglycerin for angina or inhalers for shortness of breath, due to COPD. These patients must bring these medications to their appointments and they should be readily available in an emergency drug kit.[19]
2. There are several medications that either because of the drug itself, or the condition it is used to treat, alert us to the possibility of some adverse event related to dental procedures and treatment. These would include insulin, bisphosphonates, anticoagulants, immunosuppressants, chronic steroid therapy, high-dose chronic nonsteroidal anti-inflammatory drug use and even natural drugs, such as gingko biloba and ecchinacea.[23]
3. Many medications have the potential for side effects on the oral cavity (see **Fig. 1** for the American Academy of Developmental Medicine and Dentistry Medication Dental Watch List of a list of drugs that have a direct impact on the oral cavity).[48] The most common is xerostomia, but stomatitis, gingival enlargement, and other oral pathology can arise as well. Patients must be made aware of the potential side effects and how they can minimize their risk. This can be a special challenge for those with physical and cognitive impairments that make achieving optimal oral hygiene a challenge.[23,48]
4. Even 1 prescription or over-the-counter drug can result in an adverse reaction; adverse drug interactions can occur between just 2 drugs. When prescribing medication, cross-check for possible adverse interactions. Also, review with patients the signs and symptoms of adverse drug reactions (eg, gastrointestinal upset) or potential allergy (eg, itching or rash) so that patients recognize them as early as possible.[23]

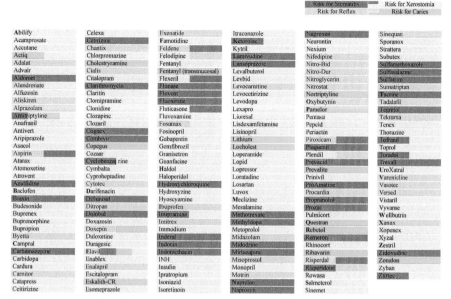

Fig. 1. Generic and trade name medication dental watch list. (*From* American Academy of Developmental Medicine and Dentistry. Generic and trade name medication dental watch list. Available at: https://aadmd.org/sites/default/files/Medication_Dental_Side_Effect_Watch_List_07-29-10.pdf. Accessed May 12, 2017; with permission.)

When there is some adverse reaction or medications do not work as anticipated and the condition does not improve as anticipated, consider the issue of compliance.[23] Many older adults may have reasons that prevent them from taking their medication or following our instructions. Ask "Why?" or "Why not?" Hearing or vision problems might result in a misunderstanding. A patient may have low literacy or low health literacy, preventing him or her from fully understanding the directions or the importance of following those directions. Others may simply be overwhelmed by the necessity of taking multiple medications or following regimens to manage their diseases.[4] They may benefit from a systematic approach or some method of reminders to take their medications correctly, such as Medisets. For those who require such measures, even the short-term medications, such as those dentists often prescribe, must be incorporated into this routine. Other patients may be dealing with issues of depression or other psychological conditions that prevent them from correctly using their medications. Others may have cognitive impairments that require others to help them safely manage their medications. In such cases, dentists should provide detailed instructions to caregivers to ensure the medications are used appropriately or consult with the patient's physician if they are uncertain about the patient's ability to manage medications.[23]

Abuse of Vulnerable Adults

Vulnerable adults are at risk of abuse and neglect. Reportedly, 10% of seniors experience abuse; however, it is largely underreported.[49,50] Abuse and neglect can be intentional (active) or not intentional (passive). Individuals, especially those dealing with depression or dementia, also can be at risk of self-neglect. See **Tables 4** and **5**,

Table 4
Victim and abuser profiles

Victim Profile	Abuser Profile
Women older than 75	Usually a relative
Lives with the abuse	Burdened by their caregiving responsibility
Dependent on the abuser	Past victim of abuse
Denies abuse	Financial dependence on the senior
Embarrassed or afraid to report the abuse	Physical or psychological conditions of their own
Fearful to report	Substance abuse

Data from Refs.[49–51]

respectively, for victim profile and abuser profile, and types of abuse and signs of abuse by type.[49–51] Note that these profiles and signs are neither exhaustive nor definitive. Practitioners should use their best judgment to determine if what they observe is likely related to some other issue, or if there is reason to suspect and report potential abuse. Practitioners may be reluctant to report suspected abuse and may be confused by signs that may be commonly associated with aging, such as bruising easily or having other trauma that patients attribute to falls or other accidents. Identification also can be a challenge for those with cognitive impairments who cannot clearly relay information.[49] Practitioners should be aware of the laws and reporting requirements in their states so that they understand expectations around reporting and how to look after the best interests of their patients. Section 3.E of the American Dental Association (ADA) Principles of Ethics and Code of Professional Conduct ADA Code states the following: dentists shall be obliged to become familiar with the signs of abuse and neglect and to report suspected cases to the proper authorities, consistent with state laws.[52]

Table 5
Types and signs of abuse

Types of Abuse	Examples	Signs: These Could Apply to 1 or More of the Types of Abuse Listed Here
Physical (includes sexual)	Inappropriate restraints, sexual abuse, deprivation of food, beating	Wounds, especially in various stages of healing
Psychological (includes verbal)	Verbal abuse, isolation, confinement	Lack of continuity with providers, that is, "doctor shopping" Reluctant or not allowed to speak for themselves
Financial	Theft, fraud, misuse of funds Embezzlement	Confusion, anger, depression, makes excuses
Neglect	Failure to assist with personal hygiene and care, failure to provide medical care or appropriate housing, directly related to the level of dependence on others for care	Lack of personal items, unpaid bills, denial of appropriate services Poor hygiene or untreated disease Isolation
Abuse by clinicians	Inappropriate use of restraints, failure to provide treatment options or coercion to accept treatment, failure to provide patient autonomy, abandonment without appropriate referral	

Data from Refs.[49–51]

SUMMARY

There are many considerations to providing safe, efficient, and appropriate care to older adults and those with special needs. Because many systemic diseases have significant direct and indirect Impacts on oral health, oral health care must be an integral component of chronic disease management. Appropriate and timely referral for oral health care from medical providers can improve overall health and wellness of patients. Dental practitioners who are not part of an established interdisciplinary care team also can reach out to other health care providers that a patient may already have to create a team.[53] This will benefit both provider and patient by expanding and integrating the resources and knowledge that is available to both. And, although it is not possible to define every older adult or individual with special needs by a single set of standards, we can use what we know about the occurrence of chronic diseases in these populations to prepare for the most likely scenarios. For those who fall outside our expectations and training, it is critical to consult with and refer to others who can help plan and provide care that is appropriate at every level of function and at every stage of life.

REFERENCES

1. Griffin SO, Jones JA, Brunson D, et al. Burden of oral disease among older adults and implications for public health priorities. Am J Public Health 2012;102(3):411–8.
2. Manski RJ, Moeller J, Schimmel J, et al. Dental care coverage and retirement. J Public Health Dent 2010;70(1):1–12.
3. Available at: https://www.cdc.gov/nchs/data/databriefs/db197.pdf. Accessed July 25, 2017.
4. Dolan TA. Professional education to meet the oral health needs of older adults and persons with disabilities. Spec Care Dentist 2013;33(4):190–7.
5. Pretty IA, Ellwood RP, Lo E, et al. The Seattle care pathway for securing oral health in older patients. Gerodontology 2014;31(s1):77–87.
6. Shay K. Identifying the needs of the elderly dental patient. The geriatric dental assessment. Dent Clin North Am 1994;38(3):499–523.
7. Kiyak HA, Reichmuth M. Barriers to and enablers of older adults' use of dental services. J Dent Educ 2005;69(9):975–86.
8. Ghezzi EM, Ship JA. Systemic diseases and their treatments in the elderly: impact on oral health. J Public Health Dent 2000;60(4):289–96.
9. Featherstone JD. Caries prevention and reversal based on the caries balance. Pediatr Dent 2006;28(2):128–32 [discussion: 92–8].
10. Young DA, Featherstone JD. Caries management by risk assessment. Community Dent Oral Epidemiol 2013;41:e1–12.
11. Young DA, Featherstone JD, Roth JR, et al. Caries management by risk assessment: implementation guidelines. J Calif Dent Assoc 2007;35(11):799–805.
12. Schwendicke F, Frencken JE, Bjorndal L, et al. Managing carious lesions: consensus recommendations on carious tissue removal. Adv Dent Res 2016;28(2):58–67.
13. Thompson V, Craig RG, Curro FA, et al. Treatment of deep carious lesions by complete excavation or partial removal: a critical review. J Am Dent Assoc 2008;139(6):705–12.
14. Twetman S, Fontana M. Patient caries risk assessment. Monogr Oral Sci 2009;21:91–101.
15. Featherstone JD, White JM, Hoover CI, et al. A randomized clinical trial of anti-caries therapies targeted according to risk assessment (caries management by risk assessment). Caries Res 2012;46(2):118–29.

16. Maeda K, Akagl J. Oral care may reduce pneumonia in the tube-fed elderly. a preliminary study. Dysphagia 2014;29(5):616–21.
17. Hurlbutt M, Young DA. A best practices approach to caries management. J Evid Based Dent Pract 2014;14(Suppl):77 86.
18. Available at: https://www.cdc.gov/nchs/data/dvs/lcwk3_2014.pdf. Accessed May 13, 2017.
19. Little JW, Falace DA, Miller CS, et al. Dental management of the medically compromised patient. 8th edition. Philadelphia: Mosby Elsevier; 2013.
20. Teeuw WJ, Kosho MX, Poland DCW, et al. Periodontitis as a possible early sign of diabetes mellitus. BMJ Open Diabetes Res Care 2017;5(1):e000326.
21. Oyetola EO, Owotade FJ, Agbelusi GA, et al. Oral findings in chronic kidney disease: implications for management in developing countries. BMC Oral Health 2015;15:24.
22. Kim IH, Kisseleva T, Brenner DA. Aging and liver disease. Curr Opin Gastroenterol 2015;31(3):184–91.
23. Chávez EM, Jacobsen PL. Pharmacology and aging. In: Pedersen PH, Walls AW, Ship JA, editors. Textbook of geriatric dentistry. 3rd edition. West Sussex (UK): John Wiley & Sons, Ltd; 2015. p. 145–54.
24. Berkey DB, Scannapieco FA. Medical considerations relating to the oral health of older adults. Spec Care Dentist 2013;33(4):164–76.
25. Kandelman D, Petersen PE, Ueda H. Oral health, general health, and quality of life in older people. Spec Care Dentist 2008;28(6):224–36.
26. Lamster IB, Lalla E, Borgnakke WS, et al. The relationship between oral health and diabetes mellitus. J Am Dent Assoc 2008;139(Supplement 5):19S–24S.
27. Chávez EM, Ship JA. Sensory and motor deficits in the elderly: impact on oral health. J Public Health Dent 2000;60(4):297–303.
28. Quandt SA, Chen H, Bell RA, et al. Food avoidance and food modification practices of older rural adults: association with oral health status and implications for service provision. Gerontologist 2010;50(1):100–11.
29. Jin LJ, Lamster IB, Greenspan JS, et al. Global burden of oral diseases: emerging concepts, management and interplay with systemic health. Oral Dis 2016;22:609–19.
30. Del Giudice A, Pompa G, Aucella F. Hypertension in the elderly. J Nephrol 2010; 23(Suppl 15):S61–71.
31. Turner MD. Hyposalivation and xerostomia: etiology, complications, and medical management. Dent Clin North Am 2016;60(2):435–43.
32. Lee JS, Kim OS, Chung HJ, et al. The correlation of carotid artery calcification on panoramic radiographs and determination of carotid artery atherosclerosis with ultrasonography. Oral Surg Oral Med Oral Pathol Oral Radiol 2014;118(6): 739–45.
33. Jacobsen PL, Chávez EM. Clinical management of the dental patient taking multiple drugs. J Contemp Dent Pract 2005;6(4):144–51.
34. Available at: https://www.cancer.gov/types/common-cancers. Accessed January 2, 2018.
35. Available at: https://seer.cancer.gov/faststats/selections.php?#Output. Accessed May 10, 2017.
36. National Cancer Institute Cancer Statistics. 2017. Available at: https://seer.cancer.gov/statfacts/html/oralcav.html. Accessed April 16, 2017.
37. Jawad H, Hodson NA, Nixon PJ. A review of dental treatment of head and neck cancer patients, before, during and after radiotherapy: part 1. Br Dent J 2015; 218(2):65–8.

38. Chung EM, Sung EC. Dental management of chemoradiation patients. J Calif Dent Assoc 2006;34(9):735–42.

39. Jawad H, Hodson N, Nixon P. A review of dental treatment of head and neck cancer patients, before, during and after radiotherapy: part 2. Br Dent J 2015;218(2): 69–74.

40. Statistics CfDCaPNCfH. COPD statistics. 2017. Available at: https://www.cdc. gov/nchs/fastats/copd.htm. Accessed April 9, 2017.

41. Rennard SI, Drummond MB. Early chronic obstructive pulmonary disease: definition, assessment, and prevention. Lancet 2015;385(9979):1778–88.

42. Available at: https://www.cdc.gov/stroke/facts.htm. Accessed January 2, 2018.

43. Mozzafarian D, Benjamin EJ, Go AS, et al, on behalf of the American Heart Association Statistics Committee and Stroke Statistics Subcommittee. Heart disease and stroke statistics—2016 update: a report from the American Heart Association. Circulation 2016;133(4):e38–360.

44. Schimmel M, Ono T, Lam OL, et al. Oro-facial impairment in stroke patients. J Oral Rehabil 2017;44(4):313–26.

45. Available at: http://www.strokeassociation.org/STROKEORG/WarningSigns/Stroke-Warning-Signs-and-Symptoms_UCM_308528_SubHomePage.jsp. Accessed January 2, 2018.

46. Available at: http://www.alz.org/dementia/types-of-dementia.asp. Accessed May 13, 2017.

47. Knoefel J, Bhaskar K. The neuropathology and cerebrovascular mechanisms of dementia. J Cereb Blood Flow Metab 2016;36(1):172–86.

48. Available at: https://aadmd.org/sites/default/files/Medication_Dental_Side_Effect_Watch_List_07-29-10.pdf. Accessed January 2, 2018.

49. McAndrew M, Marin MZ. Role of dental professional identification and referral of victims of domestic violence. N Y State Dent J 2012;78(1):16–20.

50. Evans CS, Hunold KM, Rosen T. Platts-Mills TF diagnosis of elder abuse in U.S. emergency departments. J Am Geriatr Soc 2017;65(1):91–7.

51. Available at: https://www.cdc.gov/violenceprevention/pdf/em-factsheet-a.pdf. Accessed May 13, 2017.

52. Available at: http://www.ada.org/en/~/media/ADA/About%20the%20ADA/Files/final_report_on_3e1. Accessed May 12, 2017.

53. Chávez EM, Hendre A. Caring for older adults with complex needs: drafting an interdisciplinary team. CDA J 2015;43(10):597–604.

Providing Health Screenings in a Dental Setting to Enhance Overall Health Outcomes

Barbara L. Greenberg, MSc, PhD[a],*, Michael Glick, DMD[b]

KEYWORDS

- Chairside medical screening • Diabetes mellitus • Cardiovascular disease
- Coronary heart disease • Oral health care professionals

KEY POINTS

- Chairside medical screening in the dental setting for diabetes and heart disease is effective for identifying individuals who are at increased risk of disease, yet unaware of their increased risk and who could benefit from early medical/behavioral intervention.
- Chairside medical screening in the dental setting could provide a portal of entry into the primary care system.
- Studies also suggest it is feasible to conduct these screenings in the dental setting.
- Chairside medical screening in the dental setting is viewed favorably by oral health care professionals, their patients, and primary care providers, and they are all willing to participate in such activities.
- Challenges to widespread implementation including the need for reimbursement, adequate provider training, and expansion of the state dental practice acts to include screening for increased risk of relevant medical conditions.

INTRODUCTION

Among the noncommunicable diseases (NCDs), cardiovascular disease (CVD) and diabetes mellitus (DM) continue to be among the primary causes of morbidity and mortality in the United States and worldwide. In the United States, CVD is the leading cause of death, with coronary heart disease (CHD) being the major contributor to heart

Disclosure: Neither author has anything to disclose
[a] Department of Epidemiology and Community Health, School of Health Sciences and Practice, New York Medical College, 40 Sunshine Cottage Road, Valhalla, NY 10595, USA; [b] The State University of New York, University at Buffalo School of Dental Medicine, 355 Squire Hall, Buffalo, NY 14214, USA
* Corresponding author.
E-mail address: Barbara_greenberg@nymc.edu

Dent Clin N Am 62 (2018) 269–278
https://doi.org/10.1016/j.cden.2017.11.006
0011-8532/18/© 2017 Elsevier Inc. All rights reserved.

dental.theclinics.com

disease morbidity and mortality. Diabetes is the seventh leading cause of mortality in the United States and a significant cause of morbidity,[1] Public health strategies to control these epidemics are based on preventing disease or controlling disease severity. Underlying this foundation is a focus on early disease detection and integrated health care delivery. As the health care system in the United States evolves, the emphasis on prevention and optimal health outcomes is likely to endure.[2]

Maximizing patient health outcomes will require integrated health care delivery across various disciplines. It has been suggested that the oral health care workforce could provide an additional resource in efforts to control these major health epidemics[3,4] and, accordingly, that the scope of practice for dentists be reevaluated and expanded to incorporate medical screening and primary health care activities.[5,6] In this capacity, screening is meant to be used for early identification of disease risk, which is distinct from medical disease diagnoses, which is outside the scope of practice for oral health care professionals. In many instances, patients will visit their oral health care provider on a more regular basis than a primary care provider (PCP). National Health and Nutrition Examination Survey data from 2005 showed that 54% of men who had no reported risk factors or medication use for heart disease or diabetes had not seen a physician in the prior 12 months but did see a dentist in that time period.[3] Subsequent reports using Medical Expenditure Data found that in 2008 24% of adults did not access outpatient primary care in that year, whereas 23% of those same adults did see a dentist in that same time period.[7]

Screening for the purpose of reducing a clinical outcome among individuals who have yet to develop a disease (primary prevention); screening for the purpose of reducing morbidity and mortality in an individual with already established disease, which could include disease monitoring (secondary prevention); or screening with an intent to affect the progression of an already established disease (tertiary prevention) will all require very different approaches and knowhow.[8] Furthermore, it is essential that any oral health care professional embarking on establishing a protocol for screening dental patients for systemic diseases knows what to do with any result emerging from a specific screening procedure. Screening for medical conditions in a dental setting is primarily for the purpose of identifying individuals at increased risk of developing disease based on well-established criteria, and monitoring already established disease.

Given shared underlying risk factors for oral diseases and many NCDs, such as CVD, diabetes, respiratory disease, and cancers, oral diseases have most recently been included with the NCD community (FDI World Dental Federation keeps oral health on NCD agenda),[9] and efforts to incorporate oral health within all policies are ongoing.[10] It is of interest to note that despite the plethora of studies on the associations between oral infections and systemic there is a dearth of well-designed and implemented studies elucidating the contribution of these common risk factors.[10] Such studies are necessary in order to establish optimal interdisciplinary health care delivery models. Furthermore, given the complex and often interconnected relationship among these risk factors and the likelihood of interaction across these risk factors, it is crucial that statistical analyses be appropriately conducted and interpreted to arrive at meaningful conclusions.

In this article, screening for medical conditions in the dental setting with immediate results will be referred to as *chairside screening*. Chairside screening for the presence of heart disease and diabetes has been assessed using safe, effective, and well-validated screening tools that require a blood sample for testing. Individuals found to be at increased risk of developing disease are referred to a PCP for diagnosis and determination of medical follow-up, offering dental settings to be portals for entry into the primary medical care system.[3,4]

Implementing screening for systemic conditions in a dental setting has potential value not only from a public health perspective but also as an approach to provide additional patient health-related information that could impact delivery of oral health care. Preliminary data suggest that 62% of dentists reported that screening for diabetes and CVD that yielded immediate results helped inform their treatment plan.[11]

This article presents the current state of knowledge on chairside screening in the dental setting for diabetes and heart disease risk.

PROVIDER AND PATIENT ATTITUDES ABOUT CHAIRSIDE SCREENING FOR MEDICAL CONDITIONS

Surveys in the United States have demonstrated that oral health care providers and their patients have favorable attitudes toward chairside screening for medical conditions in the dental setting.[12–14] Survey data from a nationally representative sample of practicing general dentists (N = 1945, 29% response rate, margin of error <3%) indicated that 90% of dentists thought it was important for a dentist to screen for medical conditions.[12] Among the respondents, the majority thought it was important for dentists to conduct chairside screening for each of the following conditions: hypertension (86%), CVD (77%), DM (77%), human immunodeficiency virus (72%), and hepatitis C (69%). In addition, most dentists indicated they were willing to refer patients to physicians (96%), collect saliva samples (88%), conduct screening that yields immediate results (83%), and collect finger stick blood samples (56%). Participants were also asked about potential barriers to incorporating chairside screening into their practice. More than 85% of the dentists thought that each of the issues (insurance coverage, liability, time, cost, patient' willingness) was important. The percent distribution for "very important" highlights the difference in perceived barriers; only 57% percent thought insurance coverage was "very important" compared with 75% or more for all other issues. There was no difference in the subgroup analyses for years of practice (≤10 years vs >10 years) or by gender.

A survey among a nationally representative sample of US-based practicing dental hygienists (DHs) (N = 3159, response rate 49%, margin of error <3%) found similar results to those reported among the dentists.[13] Among the DHs, 95% thought it was important for oral health care providers to screen for medical conditions; 94% thought that it was important for oral health care providers to conduct chairside screening for hypertension, 89% for DM, 85% for CVD, 79% for hepatitis infection, and 78% for HIV. As with the dentist, most were willing to refer a patient to a physician for follow-up care (94%), collect saliva samples (89%), conduct screening that yields immediate results (85%), and collect finger stick blood samples (57%). When asked about incorporating chairside screening into their daily practice activities, the most important barriers that were cited were dentist/owner support (98%), training (98%), patient willingness (98%), and time (98%). A study from New Zealand that focused on diabetes found that most general dentists participated in some aspect of disease management but were less willing to participate in hands-on activities.[14]

An equally important question is how patients feel about screening for medical conditions in a dental setting. Data from a survey among adult patients attending a university-based dental clinic or visiting dental practitioners in the community show that most patients thought chairside screening in a dental setting is important, and they were willing to participate in such activity.[15] Confidentiality was their most important concern and that the screening was not being performed by a physician was the least important. The majority thought it was important for dentists to conduct medical screening (94%) and were willing to have dentists conduct screening for CVD (81%), hypertension (90%), and DM (83%). Most were also willing to have dentists conduct screening that yields immediate results (91%), discuss results with the dentist during their visit (88%), receive a referral from the dentist to a physician (89%), provide saliva specimens (88%), provide a finger stick blood sample (75%), and pay $10 to $20 for the screening tests (69%). Most thought that if their dentist conducted these screenings, their opinion of the dentist would improve for competence (76%), compassion (76%), knowledge (80%), and professionalism (80%). In a survey of 28 dentists and 44 staff members on random blood glucose testing for DM screening in a community-based dental setting, most dentists (84%) and staff members (81%) surveyed thought "patients will benefit from blood glucose testing."[16] In the same study, 498 patients were surveyed, and most (81%) thought "blood glucose testing in the dental office was a good idea," although concern was expressed that it would be time consuming.[16]

The success of chairside screening in the dental setting requires collaboration with PCPs. Data from a national survey of PCPs (N = 1508, response rate of 22%, margin of error <3%) found the majority thought it is effective and worthwhile to conduct chairside screening to identify patients with or at risk of disease.[17] Seventy-seven percent of PCPs thought it was valuable for dentists to use screening tests with follow-up medical referral for hypertension; 71% for DM; 64% for HIV infection; and 61% for CVD. Seventy-six percent of the PCPs were willing to discuss the results with the dentist; 89% would accept a medical referral from the dentist, and 52% thought it was not important that the referral came from a dentist rather than a physician. When asked how important specified considerations would be if a proposed strategy to control disease morbidity/mortality included chairside screening by dentists with a referral to a physician for medical follow-up, 83% thought patient willingness was important, 77% thought both the level of training of the dentist and their own capacity to accept referrals was important, 66% thought duplication of provider reimbursement was important, and 58% thought duplication of roles was important.

EFFICACY AND YIELD FOR CHAIRSIDE SCREENING FOR HEART DISEASE AND DIABETES RISK USING FINGER STICK BLOOD SAMPLES

Published efficacy studies on chairside screening in the dental setting for CHD or DM were conducted and reported as early as 2007.[4] Since then, several additional studies have demonstrated the efficacy of screening for DM. The focus on screening for DM and not CHD in the dental setting is likely due to the fact that the data support a direct, synergistic relationship between PD and DM, whereas the relationship of PD and heart disease is less well defined.[18] Studies on screening for other conditions, such as obesity, in the dental setting suggest that dentists are more likely to consider screening for medical conditions for which there is supporting evidence of the oral-systemic health relationship.[19]

A screening study targeting patients (eligibility included >45 years of age; no history of heart attack, stroke, angina, or DM; not being told of any heart disease or DM risk factors; no medication use for heart disease or DM-associated risk factors; and no visit to a PCP in the last 12 months) attending in an inner-city university-based clinic was conducted to assess efficacy of chairside screening for CHD and DM in a dental setting.[4] Calibrated, trained dentists administered a CHD risk screening questionnaire, measured blood pressure, and collected finger stick blood to test for cholesterol, high-density lipoprotein, and hemoglobin A1c. Finger stick blood was used to measure total cholesterol, high-density lipoprotein levels, and hemoglobin A1c levels chairside with validated machines that yield results within 5 to 7 minutes. Clinical measurements and demographic data were used to calculate the Framingham Risk Score, which calculates the risk of a severe CHD event within 10 years. Of the 100 patients screened, 17% had an increased 10-year CHD risk (Framingham Risk Score >10%); of these, 14.0% had moderate above-average risk (>10% and <20%), and 2.2% had high risk (≥20%). In addition, 71% of participants had one major risk factor of interest, and 31% had 2 or more risk factors.[4] The recommended hemoglobin A1c cut point for abnormal A1c levels at the time the study was published was 7.0%. Using the cut point, only 1 male patient had an abnormal hemoglobin A1c level. In April 2010, the American Diabetes Association adopted a new hemoglobin A1c threshold for DM risk of greater than 5.7%; using this threshold, 21% of the patients screened in the study would have been at increased risk for DM.[20] A subsequent study in an inner-city dental school clinic looked at the efficacy of using dental features in addition to hemoglobin A1c levels for screening for DM.[21] Among adults ≥40 years of age, the data showed that A1c in conjunction with 2 dental features, at least 4 missing teeth and at least 26% of teeth with deep (≥5 mm) periodontal pockets, showed improved sensitivity for screening for DM risk. The use of hemoglobin A1c measurements alone had a 73% sensitivity, and the use of the 2 dental features alone had a 75% sensitivity for identifying unrecognized DM, whereas adding the 2 dental features increased the sensitivity to 92%.[21]

Although studies have demonstrated the yield of chairside screening in the dental setting as a means of early identification of an individual at increased risk of developing disease, it is important to assess the yield of medical diagnosis among these individuals who screen positive. A study from Sweden, a nation with a universal health care system, used the European Heart Score to identify at increased risk of dying from a CHD event within 10 years. Six percent of the individuals screened were identified as being at increased risk of dying from a CHD event within 10 years; of those who completed the medical referral, 50% were given a medical intervention.[22] A field trial was conducted in 11 general dental practices and one periodontal disease (PD) practice using hemoglobin A1c from finger stick blood to screen for metabolic syndrome and DM.[23] Among the 1022 patients screened, 41% had abnormal hemoglobin A1c values (>5.7%); of those, 35% were subsequently diagnosed with diabetes within 1 year.

Implementation of the actual screening tests in the oral health care setting is likely to be done by the DHs given their education role, and the dentist would make the final referral for follow-up medical care. A pilot study of the DHs' role in a chairside hemoglobin A1c screening protocol for diabetes among 50 patients with chronic periodontitis and no history DM found that chairside screening by DHs was effective and convenient for identifying undiagnosed diabetes.[24] Thirty-two percent of the patients had abnormal A1c levels, and there was no relationship between A1c and diabetes risk score or with other oral health indicators, including numbers of missing teeth, percentage of deep pockets, and percentage of sites with bleeding upon probing. Those who screened positive were referred to their PCP; of those, 53% contacted their PCP within 2 weeks. The direct cost of the screening was $9, and the mean screening time with discussion of results was 14 minutes. A theoretically based cost-benefit study estimated that medical screening in the dental setting for DM had the potential to save the health care system $5.1 to $65.3 million over a 1-year period depending on the rate of referral completion.[25]

More recently, studies have looked at the use of gingival curricula fluid (GCF) samples for DM risk screening in the dental setting. Data show the reliability of GCF for measuring glucose with a glucometer or self-monitoring device compared with blood glucose measurements.[26,27] In one study, a 0.986 correlation was found between GCF and with finger stick blood glucose, and a 0.972 correlation with venous blood glucose for 39 patients with DM, and 0.820 and 0.721 in 31 nondiabetic patients.[26] Another study reported a 96.7% sensitivity and 99.5% specificity for GCF compared with fasting blood glucose among 454 patients without a history of DM.[27]

CAN PERIODONTAL DISEASE STATUS SERVE AS A SCREENING TOOL FOR MEDICAL CONDITIONS?

For the past 3 decades, there has been an emerging interest in establishing an association between oral infections and overall health.[17,28] More than 3500 articles on the topic of PD and CVD, and more than 3100 articles on PD and DM, have been published since the 1940s, with more than 50% of this output having been published in the past 9 to 10 years (**Figs. 1** and **2**).

There are now a multitude of studies that have attempted to use such an association for the purpose of screening for systemic diseases and conditions, such as CVD and DM, in a dental setting. However, it is unclear if using oral diseases, such as PDs, as markers for systemic diseases and conditions, will enhance the identification of individuals with NCDs beyond what can be accomplished with using already validated risk factors and simple chairside tests for a particular systemic disease.

Nevertheless, there has been an interest among oral health care professionals to assess the predictive value of PD disease status and the possibility that it can be used as a screening tool for medical conditions such as DM and CVD. The first step is to establish if there is an independent association of PD, the medical condition of interest, and evidence that the relationship is causal. In the hierarchy of evidence, systematic reviews and meta-analysis are at the top of the pyramid and are often used to inform clinical practice guidelines and public policy. There are several issues beyond the underlying assumption that suggested guidelines for conducting meta-analyses were followed and documented and that only studies of appropriate quality were included. For example, it is essential to distinguish between studies that look at biomarkers versus hard clinical endpoints, because it is impossible to fully interpret the

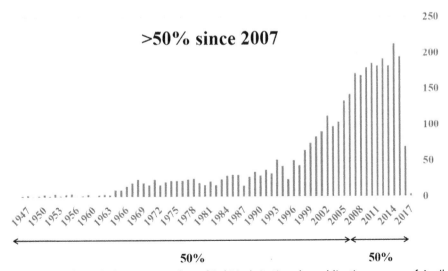

Fig. 1. PD and CVD in humans: number of PubMed citations by publication year as of April 29, 2017 (N = 3588).

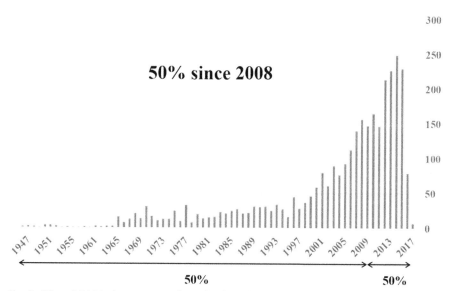

Fig. 2. PD and DM in humans: number of PubMed citations by publication year as of April 29, 2017 (N = 3161).

clinical meaning of a relationship between PD and heart disease biomarkers without clinical outcomes.

Of critical importance is also documentation of the temporal relationship between the exposure (PD) and the outcome (eg, heart disease). In order to establish that PD is in fact a risk factor that causally contributes to an incident heart disease event, it is critical to establish that the PD occurred before the heart disease. This can be particularly challenging given that both conditions are chronic with long subclinical phases. In this case, self-report of no history of heart disease is not sufficient; ideally, a cohort study included in a meta-analysis would have clinical evidence that the individuals are free of heart disease at the start of the study. Because PD is associated with known risk factors for heart disease, such as smoking, obesity, and age, it is important to determine whether potentially meaningful interactions have been assessed to more clearly elucidate the nature of the relationship. For example, is PD an independent predictor for all subgroups or only for certain age groups or only for those who are overweight? A unique challenge in systematic reviews of PD studies is the lack of a consistent and uniform definition of PD and how it is determined and operationalized.[29–31]

From an epidemiologic and statistical perspective, it is essential to consider the clinical relevance of the results. Results can be statistically significant but so small they are of little clinical or practical significance. What is considered a large enough treatment effect to make a difference should be established by the clinician and the patient and is often a subjective judgment that varies depending on the specific condition and associated consequences and potential side effects of treatment. A new treatment meant to improve PD by improving pocket depth reports a difference of 3 mm in favor of the new treatment; this difference is found to be statistically significant. Further examination suggests that a 3-mm difference is not a large enough treatment effect to be of clinical significance. Assessing study results for statistical and clinical significance is done by considering effect size and confidence intervals (CIs) around the effect size, which is beyond the scope of this article.[32]

Several systematic reviews of observational studies suggest a positive association between PD measures and the incidence of CHD.[30,33–35] Given the hierarchy of evidence in observational studies, the more important systematic reviews and meta-analyses are those for cohort studies. A meta-analysis of 5 cohort studies found that individuals with PD had a 1.14 (95% CI: 1.07–1.21) higher risk of developing CHD than those without PD.[34] A subsequent meta-analysis of 7 cohort studies found an overall risk estimate of 1.24 (95% CI: 1.01–1.51).[35] Although these results are statistically significant, based on the CIs, the question of clinical significance should be raised. Another meta-analysis that included 7 cohort studies reported a pooled risk estimate of 1.34 (95% CI: 1.27–1.42) for the association of PD and fatal and nonfatal cardiovascular events combined.[36] A more recent systematic review points out that most studies failed to show a relationship between PD and CHD in older subjects (≥65 years of age) and did not assess the relationship for other subgroups.[30] An important follow-up question to answer is whether PD has added predictive value. In one meta-analysis that did address this, PD did not improve risk prediction for heart disease beyond that of traditional risk factors.[37] As with all systematic reviews, it is important to consider the potential impact of publication bias, the fact that more positive studies get into the published literature.

SUMMARY

Data suggest that providers and patients have a favorable attitude toward chairside screening in the dental setting and are willing to participate in these activities. Likewise, efficacy studies indicate this strategy can effectively identify patients who are at increased risk of disease or have the presence of disease risk factors and could benefit from medical follow-up. Studies also suggest it is feasible to conduct these screenings in the dental setting.

Although steps have been taken to support chairside screening in the dental setting, including the establishment by the American Dental Association of dental procedure codes that could be used for screening and assessment of medical conditions, widespread implementation still faces several challenges. One of the major obstacles involves developing strategies to reimburse oral health care professionals for their time to conduct these screenings. Nevertheless, as part of an overall health care team, and in order to provide the best care to their patients, oral health care professionals may consider implementing screening protocols for medical conditions. Although this activity is still considered peripheral to the role of an oral health care provider, with the realization of value-based health care, the role of chairside screening by oral health care professionals may need to be reassessed because such screening may provide added value. The increased understanding of the relationship of oral health and systemic health may help inform optimal health care delivery both within and across disciplines. Another major challenge is the state dental boards and the reluctance of some to consider this activity within the purview of the dentist. In 2009, oral health care professionals suggested it was time to reevaluate state dental practice acts to allow for the incorporation medical screening in the dental setting as part of the scope of practice.[5,6] This issue remains a challenge today, and it is important that oral health care professionals be part of the discussions and help define what the dental practice act looks like going forward. Successful implementation will also require an appropriately trained cadre of oral health care professionals. This will necessitate integration into the dental school curricula the basics of how to conduct screenings, how to interpret and discuss the test results, when to make a referral to a medical provider, and how this information may impact oral health care delivery.

REFERENCES

1. Heron M. Deaths: leading causes for 2014. Natl Vital Stat Rep 2016;65(5):1–96.
2. Patient Protection and Affordable Care Act, 42 USC §18001–18121 (2010).
3. Glick M, Greenberg B. The potential role of dentists in identifying patients' risk of experiencing coronary heart disease events. J Am Dent Assoc 2005;136(11): 1541–6.
4. Greenberg BL, Glick M, Goodchild J, et al. Screening for cardiovascular risk factors in a dental setting. J Am Dent Assoc 2007;138(6):798–804.
5. Glick M. Expanding the dentist's role in health care delivery. Is it time to discard the Procrustean bed? J Am Dent Assoc 2009;140(11):1340–2.
6. Lamster IB, Eaves K. A model for dental practice in the 21st century. Am J Public Health 2011;101(10):1825–30.
7. Strauss SM, Alfano MC, Shelley D, et al. Identifying unaddressed systemic health conditions at dental visits: patients who visited dental practices but not general health care providers in 2008. Am J Public Health 2012;102(2):253–5.
8. Glick M. Prevention, screening and a chance of rain. J Am Dent Assoc 2015; 146(4):217–8.
9. Available at: https://www.fdiworlddental.org/news/20170213/fdi-keeps-oral-health-on-non-communicable-disease-agenda, Accessed May 29, 2017.
10. Sheihan A, Williams DM, Weyant RJ, et al. Billions with oral disease. A global health crisis - a call to action. J Am Dent Assoc 2015;146(12):861–4.
11. Greenberg B, Young M, Inge R, et al. Attitudes about chairside medical screening after conducting/receiving the tests 2016 AADR 45th Annual Meeting. Los Angeles, Calif, USA, March 13–16, 2016; 95 (special issue A).
12. Greenberg BL, Glick M, Frantsve-Hawley J, et al. Dentists' attitudes toward chairside screening for medical conditions. J Am Dent Assoc 2010;141(1):52–62.
13. Greenberg BL, Kantor ML, Bednarsh H. American dental hygienists' attitudes towards chairside medical screening in a dental setting. Int J Dent Hyg 2017;15(4): e61–8.
14. Forbes K, Thomson WM, Kunzel C, et al. Management of patients with diabetes by general dentists in New Zealand. J Periodontol 2008;79:1401–8.
15. Greenberg BL, Kantor ML, Jiang SS, et al. Patients' attitudes toward screening for medical conditions in a dental setting. J Public Health Dent 2012;72(1):28–35.
16. Barasch A, Safford MM, Qvist V, et al. Random blood glucose testing in dental practice: a community-based feasibility study from the dental practice-base research network. J Am Dent Assoc 2012;143(3):262–9.
17. Greenberg BL, Thomas PA, Glick M, et al. Physicians' attitudes toward medical screening in a dental setting. J Public Health Dent 2015;75(3):225–33.
18. Tonetti M, Kornman KS, eds. Periodontitis and systemic diseases: proceedings of a workshop jointly held by the European Federation of Periodontology and American Academy of Periodontology. J Clin Periodontol 2013;40 (suppl 14):S1–S215.
19. Curran AE, Caplan DJ, Lee JY, et al. Dentists' attitudes about their role in addressing obesity in patients: a national survey. J Am Dent Assoc 2010;141(11): 1307–16.
20. Greenberg BL. Role of oral health care professionals in overall health and well-being. In: Glick M, editor. 201A guide to patient care. The oral systemic connection. Chicago: Quintessence International; 2013. p. 1–12.
21. Lalla E, Kunzel C, Burkett S, et al. Identification of unrecognized diabetes and prediabetes in a dental setting. J Dent Res 2011;90:855–60.

22. Jontell M, Glick M. Oral health care professionals' identification of cardiovascular disease risk among patients in private dental offices in Sweden. J Am Dent Assoc 2009;140:1385–91.

23. Genco RJ, Schifferle RE, Dunford RG, et al. Screening for diabetes mellitus in dental practices. A field trial. J Am Dent Assoc 2014;145(1):57–64.

24. Bossart M, Calley KH, Gurenlin JR, et al. A pilot study of an HbA1c chairside screening protocol for diabetes I patients with chronic periodontitis: the dental hygienists role. Int J Dent Hyg 2016;14:98–107.

25. Nasseh K, Greenberg B, Vujicic M, et al. Short-term medication healthcare savings from chronic disease screenings in a dental setting. Am J Public Health 2014;104(4):744–50.

26. Parihar S, Tripathi R, Parihar AV, et al. Estimation of gingival curricular blood glucose level for screening of diabetes mellitus: a simple yet reliable method. J Oral Biol Craniofac Res 2016. https://doi.org/10.1016/j.jobcr.2016.05.004.

27. Koneru S, Tamikonda R. Reliability of gingival blood sample to screen diabetes in dental hospital. Int J Prev Med 2015;6:23.

28. Glick M, editor. The oral-systemic health connection. A guide to patient care. Hanover Park (IL): Quintessence Publishing Co, Inc.; 2014.

29. Manua C, Echeverria A, Agueda A, et al. Periodontal disease definition may determine the association between periodontitis and pregnancy outcomes. J Clin Periodontol 2008;35(5):385–97.

30. Dietrich T, Sharma P, Walter C, et al. The epidemiological evidence behind the association between periodontitis and incident atherosclerotic cardiovascular disease. J Periodontol 2013;84(4 suppl):S70–84.

31. Kelly JT, Avila-Ortiz G, Allareddy V, et al. The association between periodontitis and coronary heart disease: a quality assessment of systematic reviews. J Am Dent Assoc 2013;144:371–9.

32. Glick M, Greenberg BL. A march towards scientific literacy. J Am Dent Assoc 2017;148(8):543–5.

33. Janket SJ, Baird AE, Chuang SK, et al. Meta-analysis of periodontal disease and risk of coronary heart disease and stroke. Oral Surg Oral Med Oral Pathol Oral Radiol Endod 2003;95(5):559–69.

34. Bahekar AA, Singh S, Saha S, et al. The prevalence and incidence of coronary heart disease is significantly increased in periodontitis: a meta-analysis. Am Heart J 2007;154(5):830–7.

35. Humphrey LL, Fu R, Buckley D, et al. Periodontal disease and coronary heart disease incidence: a systematic review and meta-analysis. J Gen Intern Med 2009; 23(12):2079–86.

36. Blaizot A, Vergnes AN, Nuwwareh S, et al. Periodontal diseases and cardiovascular events: meta-analysis of observational studies. Int Dent J 2009;59(4): 197–209.

37. Helfand M, Buckley D, Freeman M, et al. Emerging risk factors for coronary heart disease: a summary of systematic reviews conducted for the US preventive services task force. Ann Intern Med 2009;151(7):496–507.

Role of Dentists in Prescribing Opioid Analgesics and Antibiotics
An Overview

Ralph Dana, DDS, MSc, FRCD(C)[a],
Amir Azarpazhooh, DDS, MSc, PhD, FRCD(C)[a,b,c],
Nima Laghapour, HBSc (C)[a], Katie J. Suda, PharmD, MS[d,e],
Christopher Okunseri, BDS, MSc, MLS, DDPH RCS(E), FFDRCSI[f,*]

KEYWORDS

- Dentistry • Dental public health • Antibiotics • Opioids • Prescription drugs
- Antibiotic stewardship

KEY POINTS

- Opioid analgesics and antibiotics as an adjunct or as a definitive treatment for common dental diseases is a useful and cost-effective measure when prescribed appropriately.
- Common dental conditions are best managed by extracting the offending tooth, restoring the tooth with an appropriate filling material, performing a root canal therapy, and/or by fabricating a prosthesis for the edentulous space.
- Appropriate and inappropriate use of antibiotics and opioid analgesics can lead to serious adverse drug events.
- Opioid analgesics prescribed as predefinitive and postdefinitive treatment for dental pain have the potential for misuse, abuse, or addiction.
- Opioid misuse and abuse are strong predictors for adverse events, including overdose.

Disclosure Statement: The views expressed in this article are those of the authors and do not necessarily reflect the position or policy of the Department of Veterans Affairs of the United States government.

[a] Faculty of Dentistry, University of Toronto, 710F-481 University Avenue, Toronto, Ontario, Canada; [b] Clinical Epidemiology & Health Care Research, School of Graduate Studies, Institute of Health Policy, Management and Evaluation, University of Toronto, 155 College Street, Suite 425, Toronto, Ontario M5T3M6, Canada; [c] Department of Dentistry, Mount Sinai Hospital, 412-600 University Avenue, Toronto, Ontario M5G 1X5, Canada; [d] Department of Veterans Affairs, Center of Innovation for Complex Chronic Healthcare, Edward Hines Jr. VA Hospital, 5000 South 5th Avenue, Hines, IL 60141, USA; [e] Department of Pharmacy Systems, Outcomes and Policy, University of Illinois at Chicago College of Pharmacy, 833 S Wood Street, Chicago, IL 60612, USA; [f] Department of Clinical Services, Marquette University School of Dentistry, Room 356, PO Box 1881, Milwaukee, WI 53201-1881, USA
* Corresponding author.
E-mail address: christopher.okunseri@marquette.edu

Dent Clin N Am 62 (2018) 279–294
https://doi.org/10.1016/j.cden.2017.11.007
0011-8532/18/© 2017 Elsevier Inc. All rights reserved.

INTRODUCTION

Opioid analgesics and antibiotics prescribed by dentists either as an adjunct or as a definitive treatment for common dental diseases is a useful and cost-effective measure when prescribed appropriately. However, many common dental conditions are best managed by extracting the offending tooth, restoring the tooth with an appropriate filling material, performing a root canal therapy, and/or by fabricating a prosthesis for the edentulous space. The appropriate and inappropriate use of antibiotics and opioid analgesics can lead to serious adverse drug events. For example, the use of antibiotics for dental infection prophylaxis has been associated with *Clostridium difficile* infection[1,2] and the development of antibiotic resistance.[3–5] Additionally, antibiotics are frequently associated with hypersensitivity reactions.[3–5] Opioid analgesics prescribed as predefinitive and postdefinitive treatment for dental pain have the potential for misuse, abuse, or addiction. Opioid misuse and abuse are strong predictors for adverse events, including overdose.[6]

Wall and colleagues[7] reported that antibiotics and pain medication accounted for 3 out of 4 drugs prescribed by dentists to patients. It is estimated that dentists prescribe about 10% of all antibiotics and opioid analgesics nationally,[8–10] and these prescriptions could contribute to the opioid analgesic epidemic, including cases of overdose in the United States.[6,11–15] Dental patients are particularly vulnerable to misuse because they regularly have leftover opioid analgesics that serve as a source for nonmedical use.[8,11–18] Persons experiencing antibiotic- and opioid-related adverse outcomes are more likely to visit the emergency department, and it is one of the leading causes of emergency department visits.[19–21] Furthermore, there is a linear relationship between inappropriate antibiotic and opioid analgesic use and adverse drug reactions.[22,23] Therefore, dentists must exercise caution in how they prescribe antibiotics and opioid analgesics. Unnecessary and excessive prescribing of opioid analgesics and antibiotics have considerable economic implications. It is estimated that treatment of opioid analgesic overdose, misuse, abuse, and diversion cost public and private insurance companies about $72.5 billion dollars annually.[24,25] Furthermore, the prescription of antibiotics is among the top therapeutic categories by expenditures in a majority of health care settings.[26,27]

Dentist prescribing practices of opioid analgesics and antibiotics have continued to receive attention from policymakers, clinicians, and patient care advocates owing to the secondary impact of these medications on population health. Unnecessary prescribing of opioid analgesics is a growing public health concern, and they are the most commonly abused prescription drug prescribed by dentists.[28] Opioid analgesic misuse often starts with either a valid opioid analgesic prescription and/or acquisition of leftover drug from a family member or friend.[6,17,18,28,29] To highlight and ascertain the state of the science of opioid analgesics in dentistry, a joint meeting was organized by the National Institute of Drug Abuse and the National Institute of Dental and Craniofacial Research.[30] At the meeting, it was concluded that data on dentist prescribing practices of opioid analgesics are scarce and that further investigations are required to better understand the role dentists play in adolescent opioid analgesic prescribing and the risk and safety associated with adolescent opioid use, as well as identifying potential roles for dentists in terms of how to prevent the opioid analgesic misuse and abuse by adolescents.[30]

Despite this meeting and seminars organized by dental professional organizations, more research is needed to demonstrate specifically the efficacy of nonopioid analgesics in the management of dental pain. In addition, innovative strategies directed specifically at dental professionals will be required to help them to reduce the prescription of opioid analgesics and antibiotics after routine dental procedures. Thus, this article highlights the state of the literature on opioid analgesic and antibiotic prescribing practices in dentistry, the impact of opioid analgesic overdose, and prevention strategies to reduce opioid analgesic and antibiotic overprescription, including public policy considerations.

OPIOID ANALGESIC PRESCRIBING PRACTICES IN DENTISTRY

Levy and colleagues[31] examined rates of opioid analgesic prescribing practices by specialty, and found that, of 4.2 billion prescriptions dispensed by US pharmacies and long-term care facilities from 2007 to 2012, 289 million (6.8%) were opioid analgesics. In addition, investigators reported that the greatest percentage decrease in opioid prescribing rates were by emergency physicians (−8.9%) and by dentists (−5.7%).[31] Rasubala and colleagues[32] reviewed data from an urgent dental center in the greater Rochester area in New York. In the study, they found that 25% of patients undergoing tooth extractions or root canal treatments received a prescription for opioid analgesics. Mutlu and colleagues[18] reported that 20% of American oral and maxillofacial surgeons prescribed excessive amounts of opioid analgesics for pain control after third molar extraction.

Pynn and colleagues,[33] in a study conducted in Canada, reported that 93% of dentist respondents prescribe an opioid for patients after removal of impacted third molars. In a more recent study conducted by Steinmetz and colleagues,[34] opioid analgesics were prescribed in 9230 dental visits (2.8%) representing more than 96 million dental visits from 1996 to 2013 in the United States. Guy and colleagues[35] reported that, nationally, rates of opioid analgesics increased from 72.4 to 81.2 prescriptions per 100 persons from 2006 to 2010, remained constant from 2010 to 2012, and then decreased by 13.1% from 2012 to 2015, but that death rates of opioid involved overdose continued to increase.[35] Despite these variations in the rates of opioid analgesic prescribing practices, the prescription of opioid analgesics by dentists is a growing public health concern. In a study based on Medical Expenditure Survey data for 1996 to 2013, investigators found an increased trend of opioid analgesic prescription after most dental procedures. Also reported were the 4 dental procedures (implants, periodontal, root canal, and surgical procedures) with the highest rates of opioid analgesics prescriptions after adjusting for patient characteristics.[34] Additionally, dental patients receive prescriptions for large doses of opioid analgesics after routine dental procedures, with limited monitoring or follow-up on how leftover medications are handled. In another study, based on the 2015 National Survey on Drug Use and Health, approximately 3.8 million people aged 12 or older reported that they misuse prescription pain relievers.[36] These are all alarming statistics and urgent attention is required to help reduce these unnecessary opioid analgesic prescription practices in the United States.

OPIOID ANALGESIC OVERDOSE, ABUSE, AND MISUSE

The World Health Organization document on the management of substance abuse describes opioid overdose as a condition characterized by a combination of 3 signs and symptoms referred to as the "opioid overdose triad."[37] The signs and symptoms are pinpoint pupils, unconsciousness, and respiratory depression. In addition, drug overdose occurs when a toxic amount of a drug, or combination of drugs, overwhelms the body.[38] The National Institute of Drug Abuse describe the misuse of prescription drugs as "taking a medication in a manner or dose other than prescribed; taking someone else's prescription, even if for a legitimate medical complaint such as pain; or taking a medication to feel euphoria (ie, to get high)."[40] In addition, according to the Centers for Disease Control and Prevention, drug diversion is when prescription medicines are obtained or used illegally by a person.[40] According to the National Institute of Drug Abuse, drug addition is a "chronic, relapsing brain disease that is characterized by compulsive drug seeking and use, despite harmful consequences. It is considered a brain disease because drugs change the structure and how the brain works. These brain changes can be long lasting and can lead to many harmful, often self-destructive, behaviors."[41]

The dentist's role in prescribing opioid analgesics is compounded by concerns for abuse, diversion and addiction. The most commonly abused opioid analgesics are immediate release (IR) agents, such as hydrocodone and oxycodone. Dentists frequently prescribe IR agents, prescribing 12% of the overall IR agents prescribed in the United States, just behind family physicians (15% of IR prescriptions).[9] Ashrafioun and colleagues[36] examined the prevalence and association of misuse of opioid analgesic prescriptions in adults seeking dental care. In the study, investigators concluded that the nonmedical use of opioid analgesics was more common in adults seeking dental care than in the general population.

According to a report published by the Centers for Disease Control and Prevention, prescription opioid overdose led to the deaths of more than 33,000 people in 2015, and this was the highest in any year recorded so far.[42] Dodd and Graham[43] reported on inappropriate prescription of analgesics for dental pain at emergency departments in the United Kingdom. On average, it is estimated that more than 1000 people are treated in emergency departments for misusing prescription opioids every day.[44–46] Some of the factors contributing to the opioid abuse epidemic include easier access to opioids within rural communities and other nonmedical sources.[34,47] It is recognized that opioids are not nearly as stigmatized or contaminated as illicit drugs, making them seem safer. In addition, health care providers have failed to anticipate the overlap between mental illness, substance abuse, and chronic pain.[34,48] Furthermore, the low cost of opioid analgesics to the insured consumer may tempt some patients to resell their medication to abusers for a large profit.[34,46] Opioid prescription misuse and abuse is a significant public health problem requiring urgent attention in the United States.[34] This crisis is receiving national attention from the media, government agencies, professional organizations, and health science research, with a focus on opioid prescribing practices, abuse, and deaths owing to overdose.

POSSIBLE ALTERNATIVES TO OPIOID ANALGESICS IN DENTISTRY

The practice of prescribing opioid analgesics for dental pain management has been based on tradition, expert opinion, practical experience, and uncontrolled anecdotal observations. Nonsteroidal antiinflammatory drugs (NSAIDs) are the preferred analgesic agent when compared with opioid analgesics, because they inhibit inflammatory reactions in addition to providing analgesia.[49,50] The effectiveness of NSAIDs in alleviating dental pain is well-established; therefore, these agents are considered to be first-line pharmacologic therapies for this indication.[49,50] In cases of severe pain where NSAIDs are not expected to be sufficient to control acute pain or are contraindicated, opioid analgesics may be considered. However, the potential therapeutic benefits of opioid analgesics must be weighed against any risks of adverse effects and narcotic dependence (which is uncommon when prescribed for no more than 3 days).[51] Recent studies have also evaluated the combined administration of ibuprofen and acetaminophen in patients who can tolerate both classes of drugs, with conclusions that this combination produces greater peak analgesia and more consistent analgesia without increasing adverse effects.[50,52,53]

Dental clinics are appropriate settings for provider and patient education on the problems associated with prescription of opioid analgesics. The management of dental pain requires that dental professionals be constantly reminded of the importance of NSAIDs as an adjunct to managing common dental pathologies. Communication among dentists, medical providers, pharmacists, researchers, professional organizations, federal agencies, and health advocates will be required for better coordination of efforts to improve dental prescribing practices of opioids.

ROLE OF DENTISTS IN THE PREVENTION OF OPIOID MISUSE

One resource available, but not frequently utilized by dentists, are prescription drug monitoring programs (PDMPs).[29,54,55] PDMPs are statewide datasets that collect data on prescriptions dispensed in a specific state for controlled substances with the highest risk of misuse (ie, opioid analgesics). Although the components of each state's PDMP differ, a PDMP generally collects information on schedule II, III, and IV controlled substances received by a patient in the past 6 months (including opioids). With these data, an individual who seeks opioids from different providers may be identified and can be prevented from receiving multiple opioid prescriptions (or other controlled substances) that may be indicative of abuse. Authorities encourage and, in some areas, mandate, prescribers to consult the PDMP before prescribing controlled drugs. However, at this time, PDMP data are not embedded in electronic health records. Thus, providers need to use a separate system to obtain the information in the PDMP.[56] Mandating use of a PDMP by dentists in New York State has been shown to reduce opioid prescriptions and increase the use of nonopioid analgesics.[32]

PRESCRIPTION OF ANTIBIOTICS IN DENTISTRY

Infection-associated inflammation is the most common cause of pain and swelling in the orofacial region. Although there is a need to treat some patients experiencing these symptoms with antibiotics, recent reports have indicated that the majority of cases do not require an antibiotic.[57] Increasing rates of bacterial resistance to antibiotics is a concern in Canada,[58] the United States,[59] and globally.[60] Recently, a National Action Plan for Combating Antibiotic-Resistant Bacteria in the United States was implemented.[61]

The global increase in bacterial resistance to antibiotics has made the management of once manageable infections difficult, extended the complexity of treatment, increased the duration of stay of patients who require hospital care, and increased the financial burden of health services.[62] The indiscriminate use of antibiotics by health care providers has been cited as one of the main contributors to the increase in and spread of antibiotic-resistant infections.[63–65] Overprescribing of antibiotics is occurring within several areas of health care in Canada,[66,67] the United States,[68–73] and has contributed to the development of antibiotic resistance and C difficile infections.[1,5]

The effect of the overprescription of antibiotics in dentistry on overall antibiotic resistance is not clear.[74] However, dentistry prescribes a considerable proportion of antibiotics (7%–11%).[4,59,75] By commonly prescribing antibiotics, the demand or expectation of patients to receive future antibiotic prescriptions negatively enforces clinicians to prescribe more to satisfy patients.[76,77] In 2014, of 31 countries, Canada ranked 12th in the outpatient antimicrobial consumption rate.[78] In the United States, a recent study estimated that nearly 30% of antibiotic prescriptions in primary care medical clinics from 2010 to 2011 were unnecessary.[79]

Treatment of common dental conditions, like all patient care, should be balanced between the need to address the patient's primary complaint and undesirable side effects of the selected treatment. Although this consideration is true of any drug prescribed by a health care provider, it is especially true of antibiotics. Despite receiving specific training regarding common dental diseases and their appropriate management, dentists are prone to prescribing antibiotics in clinical scenarios in which they are not warranted.[3,4,80-88] In fact, available cross-sectional studies have shown that dentists are likely to prescribe antibiotics when unnecessary. Some examples where antibiotics are administered inappropriately in dentistry[3,59] are as follows: lack of adherence to the current guidelines for indications of antibiotic prophylaxis; prevention of infection after dentoalveolar; periodontal or endodontic surgery; as a postoperative analgesic after endodontic treatment or for endodontic conditions without antibiotic indication; in lieu of proper drainage or after drainage without systemic involvement; for the prevention of metastatic focal infections; or to prevent claims of negligence. Various factors are hypothesized to lead to overprescribing of antibiotics, including (i) an inadequacy of the clinician's knowledge and management of patients with infectious disease, (ii) the expectations and demands of patients, (iii) a clinician's sincere desire to provide what is felt to be the "best treatment" regardless of side effects and costs, (iv) a failure to consider alternative treatments, (v) an inappropriate use of diagnostic aids, (vi) a fear of medicolegal reprimand, (vii) a belief that newer broad-spectrum antibiotics are the most effective form of treatment, and (viii) the pressures a clinician experiences in running a busy practice (ie, time and economic pressures).[58,66,89,90] Accordingly, it is not clear whether supplementing dentists' didactic knowledge regarding common dental conditions would derive a benefit in terms of reducing inappropriate antibiotic prescribing.

HOW TO IMPROVE DENTIST ANTIBIOTIC PRESCRIBING PRACTICES

Antibiotic overprescribing is a multifaceted matter. There have been multiple interventions proposed to health care professionals.[91] Interventions may include dissemination of guidelines to providers, educational meetings and lectures, audit and feedback, clinical decision support systems, mass media campaigns, and delayed prescribing.[91] Practice guidelines are controversial. Although guidelines are seen as helpful in the provision of continuing education and as a support in daily clinical decision making, the most important barrier to successful implementation of clinical practice guidelines is the fear of practitioners that guidelines will reduce their professional autonomy.[92] In fact, in a survey of dentists, only about 50% supported the development and implementation of clinical guidelines.[92] There are various barriers to the use of guidelines, even when guidelines are available.[93,94] These barriers may include a lack of awareness, lack of familiarity, lack of agreement, lack of self-efficacy, lack of outcome expectancy, the inertia of previous practice, and external barriers.[93,94] Furthermore, it has been shown that, as a standalone initiative, guidelines may not be effective unless they are specific, uncontroversial, evidence based, and require no change to existing routine.[95,96] Largely, guidelines are more effective when linked with educational initiatives.[97] Nevertheless, clear guidelines and prescribing policies should be in place as a reference standard to curtail inappropriate antibiotic prescribing practices. Palmer and colleagues[98] recommend that health care professionals need simple, clear, and practical guidelines on when and what to prescribe. Ma and colleagues[99] assessed the effect of guidelines written for physicians and patients for emergency department management of dental emergencies. Their guidelines emphasized appropriate dental clinic referrals and the use of NSAIDs. The implementation of these guidelines led to a significant decrease in visits for dental-related problems, a decrease in the proportion of patients with return visits, and a decrease in the proportion of patients receiving an opioid prescription. It is possible that guidelines may have a similar effect in reducing the antibiotic prescribing practices of dentists.

One study done in the United Kingdom by Palmer and colleagues[98] looked at whether audit, using a combination of guidelines and an educational component with feedback, could improve antibiotic prescribing among practicing general dentists. The information collected included antibiotic regimens, clinically presenting signs and symptoms, medical history, and any other reasons for prescribing before and after the audit, which included an educational component and the issuing of guidelines. After implementation of the intervention, prescriptions for antibiotics decreased by 42.5% in the postaudit period, with a concomitant reduction in the number of prescriptions that did not conform to issued guidelines.[98] This outcome suggests that audit, combined with an educational initiative and guidelines, may encourage more judicious usage of antibiotics. Another study by Steed and Gibson[100] found similar effects of audit on dentist prescribing patterns, with audit leading to a reduction in prescription writing by approximately 50%.

A study done by Seager and colleagues[101] assessed the effect of educational outreach visits on antibiotic prescribing for acute dental pain among general dentists. In this randomized controlled trial, 3 groups of dentists were randomized to standard practice, receipt of guidelines, or guidelines combined with an educational visit from a trained pharmacist. Dentists receiving the guidelines combined with the pharmacist visit prescribed fewer antibiotic prescriptions to patients with dental pain and significantly fewer inappropriate prescriptions. Interestingly, prescribing practices between the control and guideline-only groups were not significantly different. As such, it was concluded that strategies based on educational outreach visits might be successful in improving antibiotic prescribing practices among dentists.[101]

WHICH INTERVENTIONS SHOULD FUTURE POLICIES FOCUS ON?

The Centers for Disease Control and Prevention has recently established Core Elements of Outpatient Antibiotic Stewardship.[102] The 4 core elements of outpatient antibiotic stewardship are (1) commitment, (2) action for policy and practice, (3) tracking and reporting, and (4) education and expertise. Outpatient clinicians and facility leaders can commit to improving antibiotic prescribing and take action by implementing at least 1 policy or practice aimed at improving antibiotic prescribing practices. Recommended stewardship strategies may include writing and displaying public commitments in support of antibiotic stewardship, identifying a single leader to direct antibiotic stewardship activities within a facility, including antibiotic stewardship-related duties in position descriptions or job evaluation criteria, and/or communicating with all clinic staff members to set patient expectations. Possible interventions to promote appropriate antibiotic prescribing practices include the use of evidence-based diagnostic criteria and treatment recommendations, the use of delayed prescribing practices or watchful waiting, providing communications skills training for clinicians, requiring explicit written justification in the medical record for nonrecommended antibiotic prescribing, providing support for clinical decisions, and/or using call centers, nurse hotlines, or pharmacist consultations as triage systems to prevent unnecessary visits. Clinicians and leaders of outpatient clinics and health care systems can track antibiotic prescribing practices and regularly report these data back to clinicians. Clinicians can provide educational resources to patients and families on appropriate antibiotic use (ie, use effective communications strategies to educate patients about when antibiotics are and are not needed, educate patients about the potential harms of antibiotic treatment, and/or provide patient education materials). Finally, leaders of outpatient clinics and health systems can provide clinicians with education aimed at improving antibiotic prescribing and access to persons with expertise in antibiotic stewardship (ie, provide face-to-face educational training, provide continuing education activities for clinicians, and/or ensure timely access to persons with expertise).[102]

All of these interventions may be effective. The Centers for Disease Control and Prevention Core Elements recommend implementing local and/or practice-based guidelines, delayed prescribing, communication skills training, documenting a diagnosis with each antibiotic prescription, the use of clinical decision support, and educational strategies. In their 2015 systematic review, Drekonja and colleagues[103] reviewed 50 studies evaluating the effect of outpatient antimicrobial stewardship programs on prescribing, patient, microbial outcomes, and costs. They found medium-strength evidence that stewardship programs incorporating communication skills training and rapid diagnostic laboratory testing are associated with decreases in antimicrobial use, and low-strength evidence that other stewardship interventions (provider and/or patient education, provider feedback, use of guidelines, delayed prescribing, restriction policies, computerized clinical decision support, and/or financial incentives) are associated with improved prescribing practices. Although no included studies reported microbial outcomes, the few studies that reported patient-centered outcomes found no adverse effect resulting from stewardship programs. They concluded that low- to moderate-strength evidence suggests that antimicrobial stewardship programs in outpatient settings improve antimicrobial prescribing without adversely effecting patient outcomes.[103]

A 2017 systematic review focusing on the effect of antibiotic stewardship on the incidence of infections and colonization with antibiotic-resistant bacteria[104] found that antibiotic stewardship programs significantly reduced the incidence of infections and colonization with multidrug-resistant Gram-negative bacteria (51% reduction), extended-spectrum β-lactamase–producing Gram-negative bacteria (48% reduction), and methicillin-resistant Staphylococcus aureus (37% reduction), as well as the incidence of C difficile infections (32% reduction).[104] Antibiotic stewardship programs were found to be more effective when implemented with infection control measures, especially hand hygiene interventions, than when implemented alone. This systematic review concluded that antibiotic stewardship programs significantly reduce the incidence of infections and colonization with antibiotic-resistant bacteria and C difficile infections in hospital inpatients.[104] Overall, it can be concluded that there is "no magic bullet" intervention in changing physicians' prescribing habits; however, multiple interventions may lead to improved antimicrobial prescribing, without adverse effect to patient outcomes, with a reduction in the incidence and colonization of antibiotic-resistant bacteria.

DELAYED PRESCRIPTIONS OF ANTIBIOTICS

As discussed, antibiotics do not relieve dental pain, and the systemic involvement of an oral infection is the only appropriate indication for an antibiotic prescription for patients with nontraumatic dental conditions.[105] When clinicians feel it is safe not to prescribe antibiotics immediately, prescribing none with advice to return if symptoms worsen (before seeing a dental professional for definitive treatment) is an effective and prudent approach. However, in cases where the patient presents with no immediate indication for an antibiotic but where there is fear of future spreading infection or impending systemic involvement, the clinician may consider prescribing a delayed prescription of an antibiotic (ie, providing the prescription but advising the patient to delay its use for 48–72 hours in the hope that symptoms resolve or do not progress before receiving definitive treatment). A Cochrane Review that evaluated delayed antibiotics for symptoms and complications of acute respiratory tract infections found that delayed prescribing resulted in 32% of patients using antibiotics compared with 93% of patients who received immediate prescriptions (however, not prescribing antibiotics at all resulted in the least antibiotic use—14% of patients).[106] Patient satisfaction was only slightly reduced in the delayed antibiotic group (87% satisfied) compared with the immediate antibiotic group (92% satisfied).[106]

Prescribe Appropriate Antibiotic in a Sufficient Dose and at an Acceptable Duration, Only if Indicated:

The least expensive antibiotic at the narrowest spectrum of activity with the fewest possible side effects should be administered for the shortest duration in the presence of an indication (and not in lieu of a palliative or definitive treatment such as drainage) and when benefits outweigh risks. Because broad-spectrum antibiotics are more likely to lead to resistance, C. difficile, and changes in the gastrointestinal microbiota, the American Association for Endodontics recommends clinicians to use narrow spectrum antibiotics (such as penicillin VK or amoxicillin) for first-line therapy to be followed with metronidazole in case of no improvement after 2 to 3 days.[107] In penicillin-allergic patients, clindamycin should be administered.[107] Azithromycin may receive consideration as a third-line choice in those patients who are unable to tolerate penicillins or clindamycin.[107] In regard to antibiotic dosing, the Commission of the Federation Dentaire Internationale suggests that the dose of the antibiotics must be higher than the minimum inhibitory concentration.[108] In practice, antibiotic doses are targeted to be 4 times greater than the minimum inhibitory concentration.[82] When the minimum inhibitory concentration for certain bacterial strains increases, the bacteria are assigned as antibiotic resistant and standard antibiotic dosages may become ineffective to treat infections caused by the cultured organism. Removal of pathogens and/or the source of infection determines the treatment duration.[63,108] For endodontic infections, antibiotics for 5 to 7 days is generally sufficient.[3] At different doses suggested by the British National formulary, 2 to 3 days are recommended.[109,110] Prescribing antibiotics requiring fewer doses per day are more convenient for patients with improved compliance and tolerability.[109–111] To prevent microbiological and clinical relapse, antibiotics should be used for a short duration, but in an aggressive manner. Pallasch[112,113] suggests that clinicians prescribe antibiotics in sufficient doses for 3 to 5 days only, with a follow-up evaluation of the patient.

A variety of practice-altering interventions could be implemented that may subsequently curb the increase in antibiotic resistance and C difficile infections if they result in a more judicious use of antibiotics. Studies show that significant changes in prescribing habits reduces the rate at which new antimicrobial resistance accumulates.[63,75,114] Reducing antibiotic prescribing at the general practice level results in a reduced incidence of resistance in the local community, demonstrating that modifications in the prescribing habits of individual practitioners can influence the patterns of resistance.[77]

SUMMARY

Opioid analgesics and antibiotics are important pharmacologic agents available to dentists in managing common dental conditions. These agents are generally adjunctive in nature, and there is serious potential for abuse of these agents through unnecessary prescribing practices. Various interventions have been proposed to health care professionals in an attempt to curtail inappropriate prescribing practices. Dentists prescribe a significant proportion of antibiotics and opioids, and curtailing unnecessary dental prescribing can positively impact population health.

REFERENCES

1. Thornhill MH, Dayer MJ, Prendergast B, et al. Incidence and nature of adverse reactions to antibiotics used as endocarditis prophylaxis. J Antimicrob Chemother 2015;70:2382–8.
2. Thornhill MH, Dayer MJ, Forde JM, et al. Impact of the NICE guideline recommending cessation of antibiotic prophylaxis for prevention of infective endocarditis: before and after study. BMJ 2011;342:d2392.
3. Yingling NM, Byrne BE, Hartwell GR. Antibiotic use by members of the American Association of Endodontists in the year 2000: report of a national survey. J Endod 2002;28(5):396–404.
4. Dar-Odeh NS, Abu-Hammad OA, Al-Omiri MK, et al. Antibiotic prescribing practices by dentists: a review. Ther Clin Risk Manag 2010;6:301–6.
5. Cunha BA. Antibiotic side effects. Med Clin North Am 2001;85(1):149–85.
6. U.S. Department of Health and Human Services, Office of Disease Prevention and Health Promotion. National action plan for adverse drug event prevention. Washington, DC: Author; 2014. Available at: http://health.gov/hcq/pdfs/ade-action-plan-508c.pdf. Accessed February 26, 2017.
7. Wall T, Brown J, Zentz RR, et al. Dentist-prescribed drug and the patients receiving them. J Am Coll Dent 2007;74:32–41.
8. Volkow ND, McLellan TA, Cotto JH, et al. Characteristics of opioid prescriptions in 2009. JAMA 2011;305:1299–301.
9. Hicks LA, Bartoces MG, Roberts RM, et al. US outpatient antibiotic prescribing variation according to geography, patient population, and provider specialty in 2011. Clin Infect Dis 2015;60:1308–16.
10. Rigoni GC. Drug utilization for immediate- and modified release opioids in the US. Silver Spring (MD): Division of Surveillance, Research & Communication Support, Office of Drug Safety, Food and Drug Administration; 2003. Available at: http://www.fda.gov/ohrms/DOCKETS/ac/03/slides/3978S1_05_Rigoni.ppt. Accessed July 6, 2015.
11. Wright ER, Kooreman HE, Greene MS, et al. The iatrogenic epidemic of prescription drug abuse: county-level determinants of opioid availability and abuse. Drug Alcohol Depend 2014;138:209–15.
12. McCauley JL, Leite RS, Melvin CL, et al. Dental opioid prescribing practices and risk mitigation strategy implementation: identification of potential target for provider-level intervention. Subst Abus 2016;37:9–14.
13. Richard J. Durbin, United States Senator. Durbin calls on nation's medical community to curb over prescription of opioids. Available at: http://www.durbin.senate.gov/newsroom/press-releases/durbin-calls-on-nations-medical-community-to-curb-over-prescription-of-opioids. Accessed February 26, 2017.
14. Denisco FC, Kenna GA, O'Neil MG, et al. Prevention of prescription opioid abuse: the role of the dentist. J Am Dent Assoc 2011;142:800–10.
15. Porucznik CA, Johnson EM, Rolfs RT, et al. Specialty of prescribers associated with prescription opioid fatalities in Utah 2002-2010. Pain Med 2014;15:73.
16. Aldous JA, Engar RC. Analgesic prescribing patterns in a group of dentist. Gen Dent 2000;48:586–90.

17. Baker JA, Avorn J, Levin R, et al. Opioid prescribing after surgical extraction of teeth in Medicaid patients, 2000-2010. JAMA 2016;315:1653–4.
18. Mutlu I, Abubaker AO, Laskin DM. Narcotic prescribing habits and other methods of pain control by oral and maxillofacial surgeons after impacted third molar removal. J Oral Maxillofac Surg 2013;71:1500–3.
19. Shehab N, Patel PR, Srinivasan A, et al. Emergency department visits for antibiotic-associated adverse events. Clin Infect Dis 2008;47:735–43.
20. Crane EH. The CBHSQ report: emergency department visits involving narcotic pain relievers. Rockville (MD): Substance Abuse and Mental Health Services Administration, Center for Behavioral Health Statistics and Quality; 2015.
21. Budnitz DS, Pollock DA, Mendelsohn AB, et al. Emergency department visits for outpatient adverse drug events: demonstration for a national surveillance system. Ann Emerg Med 2005;45:197–206.
22. Ostini R, Jackson C, Hegney D, et al. How is medication prescribing ceased? A systematic review. Med Care 2011;49:24–36.
23. Runciman WB, Roughead EE, Semple SJ, et al. Adverse drug events and medication errors in Australia. Int J Qual Health Care 2003;15:i49–59.
24. Moghe S. Health insurance companies step up to fight opioid epidemic CNN. Available at: http://www.cnn.com/2016/05/19/health/health-insurance-companies-opioid-epidemic/index.html. Accessed July 7, 2017.
25. Katz NP, Birnbaum H, Brennan MJ, et al. Prescription opioid abuse: challenges and opportunities for payers. Am J Manag Care 2013;19(4):295–302.
26. Schumock GT, Li E, Suda KJ, et al. National trends in prescription drug expenditures and projections for 2014. Am J Health Syst Pharm 2014;71(6):482–99.
27. Suda KJ, Hicks LA, Roberts RM, et al. A national evaluation of antibiotic expenditures by health care setting in the United States, 2009. J Antimicrob Chemother 2013;68(3):715–8.
28. Substance Abuse and Mental Health Services Administration. 2012. Results from the 2011 National Survey on Drug Use and Health: summary of national findings. Available at: www.samhsa.gov/data/NSDUH/2k11Results/NSDUHresults2011.htm#Ch2. Accessed February 26, 2017.
29. Tufts Health Care Institute. The role of dentists in preventing opioid abuse. Tufts health care Institute program on opioid risk management. 12th summit meeting. Executive summary. Boston: Tufts Health Care Institute; 2010. Available at: http://www.thci.org/opioid/mar10docs/executivesummary.pdf. Accessed February 26, 2017.
30. Opioid prescribing to adolescents in dental settings. Available at: https://archives.drugabuse.gov/meetings/Dental/. Accessed July 5, 2017.
31. Levy B, Paulozzi L, Mack KA, et al. Trends in opioid analgesic-prescribing rates by specialty, U.S., 2007-2012. Am J Prev Med 2015;49(3):409–13.
32. Rasubala L, Pernapati L, Velasquez V, et al. Impact of a mandatory prescription drug monitoring program on prescription of opioid analgesics by dentists. PLoS One 2015;10(8):e0135957.
33. Pynn B, Laskin DM. Comparison of narcotic prescribing habits and other methods of pain control by oral and maxillofacial surgeons in the United States and Canada. J Oral Maxillofac Surg 2014;72:2402–4.
34. Steinmetz CN, Zheng C, Okunseri E, et al. Opioid analgesic prescribing practices of dental professionals in the United States. JDR Clin Trans Res 2017;2(3):241–8.

35. Guy GP Jr, Zhang K, Bohm MK, et al. Vital signs: changes in opioid prescribing in the United States, 2006–2015. MMWR Morb Mortal Wkly Rep 2017;66: 697–704.

36. Ashratioun L, Edwards PC, Bohnert ASB, et al. Nonmedical use of pain medications in dental patients. Am J Drug Alcohol Abuse 2014;40:312–6.

37. World Health Organization. Management of substance abuse. Information sheet on opioid overdose. 2014. Available at: http://www.who.int/substance_abuse/information-sheet/en/. Accessed July 24, 2017.

38. Harm reduction coalition. What is overdose? Available at: http://harmreduction.org/issues/overdose-prevention/overview/overdose-basics/what-is-an-overdose/. Accessed July 24, 2017.

39. National Institute of Drug Abuse. Advancing addiction science. Misuse of prescription drugs. Available at: https://www.drugabuse.gov/publications/research-reports/misuse-prescription-drugs/summary. Accessed July 24, 2017.

40. Centers for Disease Control and Prevention. Risks of healthcare-associated infections from drug diversion. Available at: https://www.cdc.gov/injectionsafety/drugdiversion/index.html. Accessed July 24, 2017.

41. National Institute of Drug Abuse. Advancing addiction science. The science of drug abuse and addiction: the basics. Available at: https://www.drugabuse.gov/publications/media-guide/science-drug-abuse-addiction-basics. Accessed July 24, 2017.

42. Center for Disease Control and Prevention. Opioid overdose. Available at: https://www.cdc.gov/drugoverdose/index.html. Accessed July 4, 2017.

43. Dodd MD, Graham CA. Unintentional overdose of analgesia secondary to acute dental pain. Br Dent J 2002;193:211–2.

44. Hasegawa K, Espinola JA, Brown DF, et al. Trends in U.S. emergency department visits for opioid overdose, 1993-2010. Pain Med 2014;15(10):1765–70.

45. Substance Abuse and Mental Health Services Administration. Highlights of the 2011 Drug Abuse Warning Network (DAWN) findings on drug-related emergency department visits. The DAWN report. Rockville (MD): US Department of Health and Human Services, Substance Abuse and Mental Health Services Administration; 2013. Available at: http://www.samhsa.gov/data/2k13/DAWN127/sr127-DAWN-highlights.htm.

46. Executive Office of the President of the United States, 2011. Epidemic: responding to America's prescription drug abuse crisis, Washington, DC. Available at: https://www.whitehouse.gov/sites/default/files/ondcp/policy-and-research/rx_abuse_plan.pdf. Accessed June 5, 2015.

47. Bohnert AS, Logan JE, Ganoczy D, et al. A detailed exploration in to the association of prescribed opioid dosage and overdose deaths among patients with chronic pain. Med Care 2016;54(5):435–41.

48. Paulozzi LJ, Weisler RH, Patkar AA. A national epidemic of unintentional prescription opioid overdose deaths: how physicians can help control it. J Clin Psychiatry 2011;72:589–92.

49. Ong CKS, Lirk P, Tan CH, et al. An evidence-based update on nonsteroidal anti-inflammatory drugs. Clin Med Res 2007;5(1):19–34.

50. Dionne RA, Gordon SM, Moore PA. Prescribing opioid analgesics for acute dental pain: time to change clinical practices in response to evidence and misperceptions. Compendium 2016;37:372–8.

51. Dowell D, Haegerich TM, Chou R. CDC guideline for prescribing opioids for chronic pain — United States, 2016. MMWR Recomm Rep 2016;65(No. RR-1): 1–49.

52. Cooper SA, Needle SE, Kruger GO. Comparative analgesic potency of aspirin and ibuprofen. J Oral Surg 1977;35:898–903.
53. Forbes JA, Kehm CJ, Gordin CD, et al. Evaluation of ketorolac, ibuprofen, acetaminophen-codeine combination in postoperative oral surgery pain. Pharmacotherapy 1989;10(6, pt 2):94s–105s.
54. Office of Substance Abuse, State of Maine. Maine's prescription monitoring program. Available at: www.maine.gov/dhhs/osa/data/pmp/. Accessed February 26, 2017.
55. Irvine JM, Hallvik SE, Hildebran C, et al. Who uses a prescription drug monitoring program and How? Insights from a statewide survey of Oregon clinicians. J Pain 2014;15:747–55.
56. Center for Disease Control and Prevention. Integrating & expanding prescription drug monitoring program data: lessons from nine states. National Center for Injury Prevention and Control. Division of Unintentional Injury Prevention; 2017. Available at: https://www.cdc.gov/drugoverdose/pdf/pehriie_report-a.pdf. Accessed July 24, 2017.
57. Longman LP, Preston AJ, Martin MV, et al. Endodontics in the adult patient: the role of antibiotics. J Dent 2000;28(8):539–48.
58. Conly J. Antimicrobial resistance in Canada. CMAJ 2002;167(8):885–91.
59. Pallasch TJ. Global antibiotic resistance and its impact on the dental community. J Calif Dent Assoc 2000;28(3):215–33.
60. World Health Organization. Antimicrobial resistance: global report on surveillance. 2014. Available at: http://www.who.int/drugresistance/documents/surveillancereport/en/.
61. Centers for Disease Control and Prevention. Committee on Antibiotic Resistance. National action plan for combating antibiotic-resistant bacteria. 2015. Available at: http://https://www.cdc.gov/drugresistance/pdf/national_action_plan_for_combating_antibotic-resistant_bacteria.pdf.
62. John JF Jr, Fishman NO. Programmatic role of the infectious diseases physician in controlling antimicrobial costs in the hospital. Clin Infect Dis 1997;24(3):471–85.
63. Ellison SJ. The role of phenoxymethylpenicillin, amoxicillin, metronidazole and clindamycin in the management of acute dentoalveolar abscesses–a review. Br Dent J 2009;206(7):357–62.
64. Sweeney LC, Dave J, Chambers PA, et al. Antibiotic resistance in general dental practice–a cause for concern? J Antimicrob Chemother 2004;53(4):567–76.
65. Antibiotic use in dentistry. ADA Council on Scientific Affairs. J Am Dent Assoc 1997;128(5):648.
66. Paluck E, Katzenstein D, Frankish CJ, et al. Prescribing practices and attitudes toward giving children antibiotics. Can Fam Physician 2001;47:521–7.
67. Wang EE, Einarson TR, Kellner JD, et al. Antibiotic prescribing for Canadian preschool children: evidence of overprescribing for viral respiratory infections. Clin Infect Dis 1999;29(1):155–60.
68. Smith SS, Kern RC, Chandra RK, et al. Variations in antibiotic prescribing of acute rhinosinusitis in United States ambulatory settings. Otolaryngol Head Neck Surg 2013;148(5):852–9.
69. Gordon LB, Waxman MJ, Ragsdale L, et al. Overtreatment of presumed urinary tract infection in older women presenting to the emergency department. J Am Geriatr Soc 2013;61(5):788–92.

70. Ackerman UL, Gonzales H, Stahl MC, et al. One size does not fit all: evaluating an intervention to reduce antibiotic prescribing for acute bronchitis. BMC Health Serv Res 2013;13:462.

71. Logan JL, Yang J, Forrest G. Outpatient antibiotic prescribing in a low-risk veteran population with acute respiratory symptoms. Hosp Pract (1995) 2012; 40(1):75–80.

72. Vanderweil SG, Tsai CL, Pelletier AJ, et al. Inappropriate use of antibiotics for acute asthma in United States emergency departments. Acad Emerg Med 2008;15(8):736–43.

73. Gonzales R, Malone DC, Maselli JH, et al. Excessive antibiotic use for acute respiratory infections in the United States. Clin Infect Dis 2001;33(6):757–62.

74. Haas DA, Epstein JB, Eggert FM. Antimicrobial resistance: dentistry's role. J Can Dent Assoc 1998;64(7):496–502.

75. Standing Medical Advisory Committee – Subgroup on Antimicrobial Resistance. The path of least resistance [press release]. London: 1998.

76. Little P, Gould C, Williamson I, et al. Reattendance and complications in a randomised trial of prescribing strategies for sore throat: the medicalising effect of prescribing antibiotics. BMJ 1997;315(7104):350–2.

77. Lewis MAO. Why we must reduce dental prescription of antibiotics: European Union Antibiotic Awareness Day. Br Dent J 2008;205(10):537–8.

78. European Centre for Disease Prevention and Control (CDC). Antimicrobial consumption rates by country. Solna (Sweden): ECDC; 2016. Available at: http:// ecdc.europa.eu/en/healthtopics/antimicrobial_resistance/esac-net-database/ Pages/Antimicrobial-consumption-rates-by-country.aspx. Accessed March 23, 2016.

79. Fleming-Dutra KE, Hersh AL, Shapiro DJ, et al. Prevalence of inappropriate antibiotic prescriptions among US ambulatory care visits, 2010-2011. JAMA 2016; 315(17):1864–73.

80. Saadat S, Mohiuddin S, Qureshi A. Antibiotic prescription practice of dental practitioners in a Public Sector Institute of Karachi. J Dow Univ Health Sci 2013;7(2):54–8.

81. Al-Huwayrini L, Al-Furiji S, Al-Dhurgham R, et al. Knowledge of antibiotics among dentists in Riyadh private clinics. Saudi Dent J 2013;25(3):119–24.

82. Sawair FA. Antibiotic prescription by general dental practitioners in the management of acute dentoalveolar infections. Saudi Dent J 2006;18(2):111–7.

83. Kumar KP, Kaushik M, Kumar PU, et al. Antibiotic prescribing habits of dental surgeons in Hyderabad City, India, for pulpal and periapical pathologies: a survey. Adv Pharmacol Sci 2013;2013:537385.

84. Vessal G, Khabiri A, Mirkhani H, et al. Study of antibiotic prescribing among dental practitioners in Shiraz, Islamic Republic of Iran. East Mediterr Health J 2011;17(10):763–9.

85. De-Bem SHC, Nhata J, Santello LC, et al. Antibiotic prescription behavior of specialists in endodontics. Dental Press Endod 2011;1(3):88–93.

86. Segura-Egea JJ, Velasco-Ortega E, Torres-Lagares D, et al. Pattern of antibiotic prescription in the management of endodontic infections amongst Spanish oral surgeons. Int Endod J 2010;43(4):342–50.

87. Rodriguez-Nunez A, Cisneros-Cabello R, Velasco-Ortega E, et al. Antibiotic use by members of the Spanish Endodontic Society. J Endod 2009;35(9):1198–203.

88. Kakoei S, Raoof M, Baghaei F, et al. Pattern of antibiotic prescription among dentists in Iran. Iran Endod J 2007;2(1):19–23.

89. Cadieux G, Tamblyn R, Dauphinee D, et al. Predictors of inappropriate antibiotic prescribing among primary care physicians. CMAJ 2007;177(8):877–83.
90. Lam TP, Lam KF. What are the non-biomedical reasons which make family doctors over-prescribe antibiotics for upper respiratory tract infection in a mixed private/public Asian setting? J Clin Pharm Ther 2003;28(3):197–201.
91. Zimmerman S, Mitchell CM, Beeber AS, et al. Strategies to reduce potentially inappropriate antibiotic prescribing in assisted living and nursing homes. In: Advances in the Prevention and Control of HAIs. Agency for Healthcare Research and Quality; 2014.
92. Van der Sanden WJ, Mettes DG, Plasschaert AJ, et al. Clinical practice guidelines in dentistry: opinions of dental practitioners on their contribution to the quality of dental care. Qual Saf Health Care 2003;12(2):107–11.
93. Birrenbach T, Kraehenmann S, Perrig M, et al. Physicians' attitudes toward, use of, and perceived barriers to clinical guidelines: a survey among Swiss physicians. Adv Med Educ Pract 2016;7:673–80.
94. Cabana MD, Rand CS, Powe NR, et al. Why don't physicians follow clinical guidelines? A framework for improvement. JAMA 1999;282(15):1458–65.
95. Grol R, Dalhuijsen J, Thomas S, et al. Attributes of clinical guidelines that influence use of guidelines in general practice: observational study. BMJ 1998; 317(7162):858–61.
96. Palmer NA, Dailey YM, Martin MV. Can audit improve antibiotic prescribing in general dental practice? Br Dent J 2001;191(5):253–5.
97. Grimshaw JM, Russel IT. Achieving health gain through clinical guidelines II: ensuring guidelines change medical practices. Qual Health Care 1994;3:45–52.
98. Palmer NA, Pealing R, Ireland RS, et al. A study of prophylactic antibiotic prescribing in National Health Service general dental practice in England. Br Dent J 2000;189(1):43.
99. Ma M, Lindsell CJ, Jauch EC, et al. Effect of education and guidelines for treatment of uncomplicated dental pain on patient and provider behavior. Ann Emerg Med 2004;44(4):323–9.
100. Steed M, Gibson J. An audit of antibiotic prescribing in general dental practice. Prim Dent Care 1997;4(2):66–70.
101. Seager JM, Howell-Jones RS, Dunstan FD, et al. A randomised controlled trial of clinical outreach education to rationalise antibiotic prescribing for acute dental pain in the primary care setting. Br Dent J 2006;201(4): 217–22 [discussion: 216].
102. Centers for Disease Control and Prevention. Core elements of outpatient antibiotic stewardship. Available at: https://www.cdc.gov/getsmart/community/improvingprescribing/core-elements/core-outpatient-stewardship.html. Accessed July 10, 2017.
103. Drekonja DM, Filice GA, Greer N, et al. Antimicrobial stewardship in outpatient settings: a systematic review. Infect Control Hosp Epidemiol 2015;36(2):142–52.
104. Baur D, Gladstone BP, Burkert F, et al. Effect of antibiotic stewardship on the incidence of infection and colonisation with antibiotic-resistant bacteria and Clostridium difficile infection: a systematic review and meta-analysis. Lancet Infect Dis 2017;17(9):990–1001.
105. Aminoshariae A, Kulild JC. Evidence-based recommendations for antibiotic usage to treat endodontic infections and pain: a systematic review of randomized controlled trials. J Am Dent Assoc 2016;147(3):186–91.
106. Spurling G, Del Mar C, Dooley L, et al. Delayed antibiotics for symptoms and complications of respiratory infections. Cochrane Database Syst Rev 2013;(4).

107. American Association of Endodontics. Antibiotics and the treatment of endodontic infections 2006. 2014. Available at: http://www.aae.org/uploadedfiles/publications_and_research/endodontics_colleagues_for_excellence_newsletter/summer06ecte.pdf. Accessed July 10, 2017.

108. Samaranayake LP, Johnson NW. Guidelines for the use of antimicrobial agents to minimise development of resistance. Int Dent J 1999;49:189–95.

109. Fazakerley MW, McGowan P, Hardy P, et al. A comparative study of cephradine, amoxycillin and phenoxymethylpenicillin in the treatment of acute dentoalveolar infection. Br Dent J 1993;174(10):359–63.

110. Martin MV, Longman LP, Hill JB, et al. Acute dentoalveolar infections: an investigation of the duration of antibiotic therapy. Br Dent J 1997;183(4):135–7.

111. Bax R. Development of a twice daily dosing regimen of amoxicillin/clavulanate. Int J Antimicrob Agents 2007;30(Suppl 2):S118–21.

112. Pallasch TJ. Antibiotic resistance. Dent Clin North Am 2003;47(4):623–39.

113. Pallasch TJ. Pharmacokinetic principles of antimicrobial therapy. Periodontol 2000 1996;10:5–11.

114. Dirks SJ, Terezhalmy GT. The patient with an odontogenic infection. Quintessence Int 2004;35(6):482–502.

Trends in Pediatric Dental Care Use

Natalia I. Chalmers, DDS, PhD[a],*, Joseph S. Wislar, MS[b], Matt Hall, PhD[c],
Cary Thurm, PhD[c], Man Wai Ng, DDS, MPH[d]

KEYWORDS

- Pediatric oral health • Health disparities • Emergency department • Operating room
- Medicaid EPSDT Benefit

KEY POINTS

- Small increases in reimbursement, in states with fewer dentists and with low Medicaid participation, can increase use of prevention and diagnostic services.
- Most children receiving treatment in the operating room (OR) for dental conditions are healthy. Children with complex chronic conditions are more likely to return for OR treatment.
- Patients aged 19 to 20 years have the highest emergency department (ED) rates for dental conditions. For all ages, visits to the ED for preventable dental conditions are decreasing.
- Early access to preventive dental services together with care coordination for Medicaid-eligible children can prevent the costly treatment of dental conditions in hospital ORs and EDs.

INTRODUCTION

There is a significant shift in health care from volume to value, and dentistry has a tremendous challenge and an opportunity in this shift. The cost of care and limited access to care remain significant barriers.[1,2] Addressing the rapidly increasing costs of care, increasing access to care, and improving oral health outcomes will require the simultaneous pursuit of 3 aims: (1) improving the care experience, (2) improving the health of populations, and (3) reducing per capita costs of health care.[3]

National health expenditure projections for dental services will reach $185.0 billion in 2025.[4] This significant spending has not translated to better access or patient outcomes because 23% of children continue to have dental caries, with children 2 to 5 years old experiencing increasing rates.[5] Also, the United States spent $26.5 billion

Funding Sources: None.
Disclosures: None.
[a] Analytics and Publication, DentaQuest Institute, 10320 Little Patuxent Parkway, Suite 214, Columbia, MD 21044, USA; [b] Analytics and Publication, DentaQuest Institute, 10320 Little Patuxent Parkway, Suite 214, Columbia, MD 21044, USA; [c] Children's Hospital Association, 600 13th Street NW, Washington, DC 20005, USA; [d] Department of Pediatric Dentistry, Boston Children's Hospital, 300 Longwood Avenue, Boston, MA 02115, USA
* Corresponding author.
E-mail address: Natalia.Chalmers@DentaQuestInstitute.org

0011-8532/18/© 2017 The Authors. Published by Elsevier Inc. This is an open access article under the CC BY-NC-ND license (http://creativecommons.org/licenses/by-nc-nd/4.0/).

for dental services for children less than age 21 years in 2013[6]. What is not reflected in this number is the significant additional cost burden that the health care system experiences for dental and oral health encounters in expensive settings such as emergency departments (EDs) and operating rooms (ORs).

This article explores trends in 3 areas of dental services use for children less than 21 years of age. First, it examines the change in access to prevention, diagnostic, and treatment services over time among Medicaid-enrolled children and how access to care is affected by state-level factors. Second, it evaluates trends and health care costs associated with the treatment of oral health conditions in the ORs of pediatric hospitals. Third, it examines the trends in use of EDs for dental and oral health diagnoses among children less than age 21 years in the United States.

Limited access to care can lead to postponing of preventive and surgical dental care, which in turn can result in seeking care in an ED setting. If the disease state is advanced, dental treatment in the OR may be required. Addressing the silent epidemic of poor oral health[7] will not require more spending but better spending. Dental caries is a chronic disease that is significantly influenced by social and behavioral factors but that is also largely preventable. Improving access to and the use of prevention and disease management strategies, along with early preventive dental visits, can be expected to lead to better patient outcomes, reduction of per capita health care expenses, and improved access to preventive and treatment services.

PART 1: TRENDS IN ACCESS TO DENTAL SERVICES (PREVENTION, TREATMENT, DIAGNOSIS) BY STATE AND AGE

The Early and Periodic Screening, Diagnostic, and Treatment (EPSDT) program was created in 1967 as a means to combat the effects of poverty on the health of children.[8] This preventive services benefit program is mandated for children receiving Medicaid, but there is variability by states in the application of the EPSDT guidelines.[9] Although the EPSDT services are mandated, access through provider participation in Medicaid is not guaranteed.[10]

With a significant number of new children becoming eligible, the authors think there is a need to clearly define 2 concepts. The first is access to the health care delivery system; that is, of those children who are eligible, how many can connect with and access dental services. The second concept is the type of care children received once they have access to the health care system; that is, of the children who have access to the health care delivery system, how many receive prevention, treatment, and diagnostic services. The first concept addresses the capacity of the system to accommodate the eligible beneficiaries, whereas the second concept addresses the type of care children receive once they have successfully connected with the delivery system.

Some research suggests that Medicaid reimbursement rates may affect patient access to the dental care delivery system by increasing dentist participation in the Medicaid program.[10–14] Previous research has also shown that the relationship between Medicaid reimbursement rates and access to dental care is moderated by both dentist geographic density and by the proportion of dentists participating in the Medicaid program.[10] Access to dental services may be reduced in those states that have low dentist geographic density and low rates of provider participation in the Medicaid program, but it has not previously been shown how these factors may affect access to treatment and diagnostic services. Furthermore, the effect of differential access rates by age groups remains unexplored.

The access to prevention, diagnostic, and treatment services are described here as a rate of all who are eligible, and this article further focuses on the ratio of children who receive these services to those who have access to the system. State-level factors that may affect access to the oral health care delivery system are also examined.

Methods

The data for the study were extracted from the Centers for Medicare & Medicaid Services (CMS)-416 EPSDT report for states' Medicaid and CHIP programs' effectiveness from 2010 to 2015. Reporting includes the numbers of children who were (1) provided with health screening services, (2) referred for treatment, and (3) received dental services. The CMS-416 data used in the current analysis include 50 US states and the District of Columbia for all children 0 to 20 years of age, stratified by 7 age categories.

Using these data, the authors created 2 types of indices: rate (access to prevention, diagnostic, and treatment services) and a ratio (receipt of prevention, diagnostic, and treatment). Rates measure the access to dental care and services as a percentage of children with at least 90 days of continuous Medicaid coverage eligible to receive a service. Ratios measure the dental services received as a percentage of children who obtained at least 1 dental service and thus used the oral health delivery system; that is, the eligible children who have received at least 1 dental service in the previous year (Appendix 1 provides details on rate calculations, variables, and methods used).

To further understand the impact of state-level factors on the rates of access, linear regression models were developed for 2014 to test the relationships between state-level factors and dental service use as measured by our indices. We considered several variables as potential mediators and/or moderators in the reimbursement and service use pathway. First, we estimated the effect of Medicaid reimbursement, as percent of the commercial plan at the state level.[15] Second, we included 2 measures of dentist density: the number of professionally active dentists per 100,000 population in 2014, and the percentage of dentists participating in Medicaid for child services in 2014 (participation rate).[15–17] To account for potential confounding effects, we included, as risk adjustment factors, median household income, extracted from the American Community Survey, and the Oral Health Index (OHI) as a measure of the state dental quality ranking. The OHI was developed by WalletHub using 23 weighted state-level metrics totaling 100 points.[18] Higher scores indicate more favorable conditions for oral health (Appendix 2 provides data).

A nested model-building approach was used to test relationships between these variables. First, main effects models were constructed to include reimbursement rates, density measures, household income, and OHI. Then, 2-way and 3-way interaction terms were tested between the dentist and Medicaid variables. In the interest of space, and to be consistent with our previous research, this article only discusses the 3-way interaction models, but all model results (main effects, 2-way, and 3-way interactions) are available in Appendix 3. We did not adjust for multiple comparisons.

Results

Trends in rates and ratios

Rates and ratios over time for all groups from 2010 to 2015 are shown in **Fig. 1**.

Combining all age groups (see **Fig. 1A**), rates of access to services are generally lower than ratios of receiving services. This finding indicates that eligible children have some difficulty accessing dental care but, once they have successfully navigated the care delivery system, they receive at least 1 preventive, diagnostic, and treatment service. Access, prevention, and diagnostic service rates and ratios have been steadily increasing, whereas the treatment rates and ratios have declined slightly over time. Access to, and use of, preventive and diagnostic dental care is lowest among children less than 1 year of age (see **Fig. 1B**). There are steady increases for

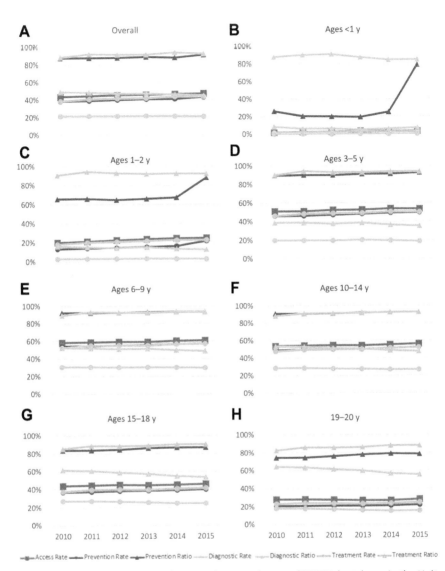

Fig. 1. Rates of access and ratios of services for several types of EPSDT dental care in the United States, 2010 to 2015. (*Data from* Centers for Medicaid and Medicare Services. EPSDT data. Available at: https://www.medicaid.gov/medicaid/benefits/epsdt/index.html. Accessed March 29, 2017.)

ages 1 to 2 years (see **Fig. 1**C) and 3 to 5 years (see **Fig. 1**D), and peaks among those aged 6 to 9 years (see **Fig. 1**E), before declining again for children aged 10 to 14 years (see **Fig. 1**F), 15 to 18 years (see **Fig. 1**G), and 19 to 20 years (see **Fig. 1**H). The large spike in the prevention ratio among those 2 years of age and younger in 2015 is in part caused by the establishment of the First Dental Home program in Texas.[19] Although access to treatment services follows a similar pattern, the ratio of treatment services to all those receiving dental care is highest among older children.

National trends can mask wide variation between states. **Fig. 2** shows the state-by-state variation in 2014 for the rates included in these analyses. The access rate for the United States was 47.6% but showed wide state-by-state variability, with Connecticut

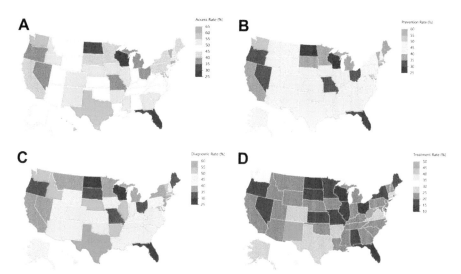

Fig. 2. EPSDT dental care services use rates for Medicaid-eligible children in the United States, 2014. (*Data from* Centers for Medicaid and Medicare Services. EPSDT data. Available at: https://www.medicaid.gov/medicaid/benefits/epsdt/index.html. Accessed March 29, 2017.)

reporting the highest rate of access to dental services (62.0%) and Wisconsin reporting the lowest (27.4%; see **Fig. 2**A). The prevention rate was 43.5% nationally but was highest in Vermont (59.6%) and lowest in Wisconsin (25.0%; see **Fig. 2**B). The diagnostic rate for the United States as a whole in 2014 was 44.1%, suggesting that less than half of eligible children who saw a dentist received diagnostic services. However, this rate ranged from 25.3% in Wisconsin to 58.6% in Texas (see **Fig. 2**C). The treatment rate was 22.4% nationally but varied from the highest in New Mexico (49.9%) to a low in Wisconsin (10.9%; see **Fig. 2**D).

Access rate to dental services

Here the access and prevention services rates by the 7 CMS-416 age groups are reported. The 3-way interaction access rate models were consistent across 6 of the 7 age categories and were similar to the model including all ages (see panel A, Appendix 3). The significant interaction terms suggest that the relationship between state reimbursement rates and the access rate was moderated by the dentist density indices. However, an increase in the reimbursement rate may not have an impact on access for the oldest youth who are eligible for EPSDT services. Income and OHI had negligible impacts beyond the effects of density, reimbursement, and participation rates already discussed.

To illustrate the interpretation of this small, but significant, interaction term, this article includes **Table 1** with data from the all-ages model. In states with average to high dentist density, the model predicted an increase in the access rate of between 0.27% (low participation states) and 0.52% (high participation states) for every 1% increase in the Medicaid reimbursement rate. Dentist density was important as well. Low-density states with low participation rates reported nearly a 1.0% higher access rate (0.95%). There is no effect of reimbursement rate when states had low dentist density combined with high participation in Medicaid.

Prevention services rate

Like the access rate models, the models predicting prevention rates were remarkably similar across all age categories (see panel B, Appendix 3). The interactive effect of

Table 1
Linear predictions from interaction terms in regression models estimating effect of Medicaid reimbursement rates on Early and Periodic Screening, Diagnostic, and Treatment service rates in the United States (all ages)

Panel A: Access Rate

| | Slope of Linear Prediction of Reimbursement Rate in 2013 | | Difference in Slopes | | | | | |
| | | | Vs Low Dentist Density, High Medicaid Dentist Density | | Vs High Dentist Density, Low Medicaid Dentist Density | | Vs High Dentist Density, High Medicaid Dentist Density | |
	Slope	SE	Difference	T Value	Difference	T Value	Difference	T Value
Low Dentist Density, Low Medicaid Dentist Density	0.95[a]	0.33	−1.22[a]	3.05	−0.68[a]	2.74	−0.43[a]	2.01
Low Dentist Density, High Medicaid Dentist Density	−0.28	0.28	—	—	0.55[a]	1.99	0.80[a]	2.13
High Dentist Density, Low Medicaid Dentist Density	0.27[a]	0.09	−0.55[a]	1.99	—	—	0.25	1.85
High Dentist Density, High Medicaid Dentist Density	0.52[a]	0.19	−0.80[a]	2.13	−0.25	1.85	—	—

Panel B: Prevention Services Rate

| | Slope of Linear Prediction of Reimbursement Rate in 2013 | | Difference in Slopes | | | | | |
| | | | Vs Low Dentist Density, High Medicaid Dentist Density | | Vs High Dentist Density, Low Medicaid Dentist Density | | Vs High Dentist Density, High Medicaid Dentist Density | |
	Slope	SE	Difference	T Value	Difference	T Value	Difference	T Value
Low Dentist Density, Low Medicaid Dentist Density	1.02[a]	0.29	−1.18[a]	3.26	−0.72[a]	2.60	−0.55[a]	2.13
Low Dentist Density, High Medicaid Dentist Density	−0.16	0.22	—	—	0.46[a]	1.95	0.63[a]	2.01
High Dentist Density, Low Medicaid Dentist Density	0.30[a]	0.12	−0.46[a]	1.95	—	—	0.17	1.51
High Dentist Density, High Medicaid Dentist Density	0.47[a]	0.16	−0.63[a]	2.01	−0.17	1.51	—	—

Panel C: Diagnostic Services Rate

| | Slope of Linear Prediction of Reimbursement Rate in 2013 | | Difference in Slopes | | | | | |
| | | | Vs Low Dentist Density, High Medicaid Dentist Density | | Vs High Dentist Density, Low Medicaid Dentist Density | | Vs High Dentist Density, High Medicaid Dentist Density | |
	Slope	SE	Difference	T Value	Difference	T Value	Difference	T Value
Low Dentist Density, Low Medicaid Dentist Density	0.96[a]	0.26	-1.15[a]	3.16	-0.72[a]	2.62	-0.44[a]	2.01
Low Dentist Density, High Medicaid Dentist Density	-0.18	0.20	—	—	0.42[a]	1.92	0.71[a]	2.15
High Dentist Density, Low Medicaid Dentist Density	0.24[a]	0.11	-0.42[a]	2.01	—	—	0.29	1.79
High Dentist Density, High Medicaid Dentist Density	0.53[a]	0.16	-0.71[a]	2.15	-0.29	1.79	—	—

Note: high density is 1 standard deviation greater than the mean and low density is 1 standard deviation less than the mean. Interaction terms were not significant for the treatment service rate, so this table was not generated.

Abbreviation: SE, standard error.

[a] P<.05.

Data from Centers for Medicaid and Medicare Services. EPSDT data. Available at: https://www.medicaid.gov/medicaid/benefits/epsdt/index.html. Accessed March 29, 2017.

reimbursement rates, participation rates, and dentist density was again small, but significant, in each model except for individuals 19 to 20 years old. These differences are highlighted in **Table 1**. In states with average to high dentist density, the model predicted an increase in the prevention services rate of between 0.30% and 0.47% for every 1% increase in the reimbursement rate depending on level of dentists participating in Medicaid. However, in low-density states with low provider participation in Medicaid, there was a 1.02% higher prevention services rate, but a nonsignificant change in the rate for states with the combination of low density and high participation. This finding suggests that small increases in the reimbursement rate would have a modest improvement effect on the receipt of preventive dental services for most children living in states with high dentist density. In addition, children living in low-density and low-participating states may receive an even larger boost in preventive services with an increase in Medicaid reimbursement rates.

Diagnostic services rate

Panel C in Appendix 3 shows the 3-way interaction models for diagnostic services rates. There are significant interactive effects across all age categories except for the youngest and oldest. These findings follow clinical expectations in that children less than 1 year old are unlikely to need diagnostic services and are thus unlikely to be affected by changes in reimbursement or participation rates. In contrast, the oldest youth may be less influenced by state-level factors given their increased independence, mobility, and decision-making capabilities.

As with the access and prevention rate models, the significant interaction term suggests that the relationship between the reimbursement and diagnostic services rates was moderated by the 2 density measures. The differences in these slopes for all ages combined are shown in **Fig. 3** and **Table 1** and are very similar to the access rate model. For example, in states with average to high dentist density, the model predicted an

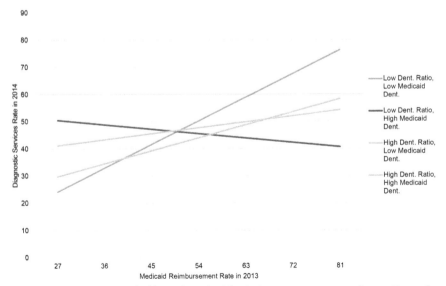

Fig. 3. Linear prediction of effect of Medicaid reimbursement rate on diagnostic services rate, by dentist density (Dent.) and dentists participating in Medicaid. (*Data from* Centers for Medicaid and Medicare Services. EPSDT data. Available at: https://www.medicaid.gov/medicaid/benefits/epsdt/index.html. Accessed March 29, 2017.)

increase in the diagnostic services rate of between 0.24% and 0.53% for every 1% increase in the reimbursement rate depending on level of Medicaid participation. However, in low-density states with low participation, there was nearly a 1.0% higher diagnostic rate (0.96%), and a nonsignificant slope for low-density states with high participation.

Treatment services rate

The models predicting treatment service rates are shown in panel D (see Appendix 3). None of the 3-way interaction terms were significant for any age group. However, the main effects models showed associations between reimbursement rates and dentist density for all age groups 3 to 5 years old and older. For example, in the main effects model including all ages, every 1% increase in reimbursement is associated with a 0.21% increase in treatment. Likewise, an increase in dentist density was associated with a 0.33% increase in treatment services provided.

Discussion

Addressing the access gap for dental care is not as simple as only increasing the reimbursement fees. The presented findings from the models suggest there is evidence for a mediating relationship between Medicaid reimbursement rates and the use of dental services through rates of dentist participation in Medicaid, with little variability by patient age. Dentist density indicators moderated the relationship between Medicaid reimbursement rates and access to services, but not treatment. In states with average or high dentist densities, there was a moderate and positive relationship between Medicaid reimbursement rates and use of services. In those states, the proportion of dentists accepting Medicaid had little impact. In states with low dentist densities and fewer dentists participating in Medicaid, higher reimbursement rates were associated with significantly better dental services use. In states with low dentist densities but high participation in Medicaid, reimbursement rates had no effect.

Our models suggest that the reimbursement rates affect getting eligible children to the dental office but not the services received once there. The models also suggest that an increase in the reimbursement fee in itself does not help in getting more of the youngest eligible children into the dental office, but it does help the older youth.

Similar to the authors previous research, the authors can identify potential pathways to increased access to dental care, prevention, diagnostics, and treatment. In states with fewer dentists and with low participation in Medicaid, even small increases in reimbursement rates may yield large effects on access to dental care and, likewise, use of prevention and diagnostic services. States with average or high numbers of dentists may also benefit from increasing reimbursement rates, although these benefits may not be as noteworthy. In contrast, it is possible that states with fewer dentists but high rates of Medicaid participation may not see much benefit from increasing reimbursement rates.

PART 2: USE OF OPERATING ROOMS FOR TREATMENT OF DENTAL CONDITIONS

Earlier in this article it was shown that access to care can be affected by state-level factors even though coverage is mandated. Despite that mandate, access to dental caries management remains limited for Medicaid-enrolled children.[20] In 2015, 57% of Medicaid children nationally received no preventive dental services (see **Fig. 1**A). The lack of preventive care may contribute to an increased risk of dental caries and other preventable conditions. Young children and individuals with special health care needs with dental caries commonly require dental treatment under general anesthesia (GA), often in hospital ORs, which are some of the costliest settings in which to deliver dental care.

Need for Care in the Operating Room

Dental caries is the primary diagnosis for two-thirds of ambulatory surgery visits by children younger than 6 years, with 3-year-olds having the highest rate of hospitalization for caries treatment.[21] According to the American Academy of Pediatric Dentistry, the use of GA is sometimes necessary to provide quality care for the child.[22,23] This type of care can be provided in a hospital or an ambulatory setting, such as the dental office[22] or an ambulatory surgery center.[24]

Chronic conditions (episodic/lifelong/complex) can affect the need for dental treatment under GA, especially in Medicaid-enrolled children between the ages of 8 and 14 years.[25] Children with special health care needs often require advanced behavioral guidance for the management of early childhood caries (ECC). The most common specific underlying diagnoses in one study were autism (38%), cerebral palsy/developmental delay (18%), and attention-deficit/hyperactivity disorder (4%).[26]

Additional evidence suggests that the treatment intensity index (TII), a weighted sum of the types of dental services performed, differs significantly between children treated in the OR and those treated in non-OR settings, with children treated under GA having a higher TII.[27]

Cost of Dental Care in the Operating Room

Treatment of dental caries in Medicaid children in the hospital setting creates a large expense burden for the health care system. For example, research from the mid-1990s in Louisiana showed that the cost of providing dental care in hospitals to children 1 to 5 years old accounted for 45% of the total dental costs, even though this age group only comprised 5% of the insured population.[27] The high cost for this age group came from the dental treatment provided to them in the OR. The mean cost of care provided to children in the OR was 14.5 times higher for children treated elsewhere.[27] Another study found that 9% of Medicaid-enrolled children with high dental expenses (>$1000/y) incurred 64% of total dental costs.[28] A related study found that fewer than 2% of Medicaid-enrolled children less than 6 years of age accounted for 25% of all dollars spent on dental services for this age group.[29]

Ambulatory surgery centers are emerging as an alternative to hospital-based settings where children with dental conditions can be treated. Only 1% of children enrolled in Medicaid received dental care in these settings in 2011, with average costs much lower than for the OR.[24] Recent chronic disease management (CDM) programs designed to prevent the occurrence and recurrence of ECC shows the cost-effectiveness of these programs and their potential to reduce health care costs significantly.[30]

Treatment Outcomes in the Operating Room

Children with ECC may become malnourished and fail to thrive as a result of having oral pain and infection, which can alter eating and sleeping patterns. After undergoing comprehensive dental rehabilitation in the OR under GA, these children show improvements in both weight and growth.[31] In addition, the quality of life for children and their caregivers can significantly improve after dental rehabilitation in the OR.[32] However, because of the advanced state of the disease at the time of rehabilitation, most children require the extraction of between 1 and 6 teeth. Extractions are then associated with increased fear following the rehabilitation.[32] The impact of severe ECC can be so grave that 3-year-old children may require full dentures.[33]

Although GA provides an optimal condition for treating children with high caries risk, high rates of new and recurrent caries develop nevertheless.[34–37] Caries is an infectious disease, and antimicrobial interventions and treatments, including dental rehabilitation under GA, for ECC show only temporary reductions (3 months) in *Streptococcus mutans* colonization levels.[38] This finding suggests that achieving sustainable effects on cariogenic microbial colonization and ECC reduction will require alternative prevention strategies.[39]

Composite restorations done under GA can show high failure rates.[40] One study showed a high failure rate (50%) of amalgam or composite restorations.[41] Placement of stainless steel crown (SSC) is the most frequently performed procedure,[21] with an average of 6 SSCs per case in some studies.[29] Because of the high initial costs of treating ECC under GA, it is preferable that both the short-term and long-term longevity of restorative treatments be optimized.

A descriptive analysis of patients treated for dental caries under GA in pediatric hospitals is presented later.

Methods

In this retrospective, multicenter, longitudinal analysis, the authors used administrative data from the Pediatric Health Information System (PHIS) to assess OR use for oral health–related conditions. Forty-five children's hospitals report to PHIS. We extracted data on pediatric patients (aged 1–20 years) with 1 or more visits to the OR for a dental or oral health–related condition (DOHRC) diagnosis between 2010 and 2012. Patients were followed for 3 years after their initial OR visit. Visits were identified using The International Classification of Diseases, Ninth Revision, Clinical Modification (ICD-9-CM) procedure codes 521.0 through 529.9. In the literature, these are sometimes referred to as nontraumatic dental conditions. The pediatric complex chronic conditions (CCC) classification system was used to identify children with ($\geq$1 CCC) and without CCC.[42]

Results

During the study period, 55,740 children received treatment in the OR for dental conditions (**Table 2**). Most (82.6%) of these children had no CCC and 94.3% of patients only had a single visit. However, children with CCC were much more likely to return to the OR. Only 3.8% of children without CCC had multiple OR visits in the 3-year study period compared with 15.0% of children with CCC.

Patients with multiple OR visits had much higher cost burdens ($28.9 million; 15% of the total spent on 5.7% of patients) than those with a single visit ($162 million; 85% of the total spent on 94.3% of patients). Patients with 1 or more CCC had even higher cost burdens for repeat OR visits ($16.4 million; 8.6% of the total spent to treat 2.6% of all patients).

Discussion

As stated earlier, children with special health care needs may need advanced behavior modification or other specialized care, thus requiring dental care in the OR.[21] Our findings show that most of the children treated in the OR for dental needs do not have a complex chronic condition. Because these potentially unnecessary OR visits at children's hospitals generate a substantial cost burden, alternative, less costly models for treatment of healthy children for dental caries are needed.

Disease management

Considering the significant costs associated with dental rehabilitation under GA in the OR, along with the high rates of new and recurrent caries after the dental rehabilitation, new strategies are needed beyond the traditional restorative and surgical approaches currently used in children. CDM is a risk-based approach based on Wagner's chronic

Table 2
Patients aged 0 to 20 years with an operating room visit related to a dental or oral health–related condition between 2010 and 2012

	Number of Visits							
	Overall		No CCC Present			CCC Present		
Visits (n)	Count	%	Count	% with No CCC	% of Overall	Count	% with CCC	% of Overall
1	52,548	94.3	44,283	96.2	79.4	8265	85.0	14.8
2	2620	4.7	1547	3.4	2.8	1073	11.0	1.9
3	382	0.7	144	0.3	0.3	238	2.4	0.4
4+	190	0.3	46	0.1	0.1	144	1.5	0.3
Total	55,740	100.0	46,020	100.0	82.6	9720	100.0	17.4

	Costs							
	Overall		No CCC Present			CCC Present		
Visits (n)	Count ($)	%	Count ($)	% with No CCC	% of Overall	Count ($)	% with CCC	% of Overall
1	162,181,810	84.9	128,480,895	91.1	67.2	33,700,916	67.2	17.6
2	19,347,403	10.1	10,139,948	7.2	5.3	9,207,456	18.4	4.8
3	5,009,971	2.6	1,607,155	1.1	0.8	3,402,817	6.8	1.8
4+	4,594,544	2.4	730,368	0.5	0.4	3,864,176	7.7	2.0
Total	191,133,728	100.0	140,958,366	100.0	73.7	50,175,365	100.0	26.3

Note: DOHRCs are defined as diagnoses of ICD-9-CM codes 520.0 through 529.9.
Data from Children's Hospital Association. Pediatric Health Information System. Available at: https://www.childrenshospitals.org/programs-and-services/data-analytics-and-research/pediatric-analytic-solutions/pediatric-health-information-system. Accessed June 8, 2016.

care model.[43] In CDM, the professional care team aims to help patients and their families effectively manage their own disease using reliable, evidence-based practices.[43]

CDM assumes that caries is a dynamic process that can be controlled by addressing the caries balance through the control of risk factors and augmentation of protective factors. Health care providers help their patients with self-management through coaching and encouragement to alter lifestyle behaviors (dietary and oral hygiene practices) and improve their health outcomes. CDM moves beyond education to empowering patients to take control of their own health and focuses on helping patients and their families to effectively manage their own disease. Frequent caries risk assessment, revision of self-management goals, caries charting to document disease status and activity, use of remineralization strategies such as fluorides (fluoride toothpastes, fluoride varnish, silver diamine fluoride), xylitol and casein phosphate products, sealants, interim restorative treatment and conventional restorative treatment, and recare based on caries risk are components of the CDM protocol.[44]

Early results of CDM endeavors to address ECC have shown a reduction in caries incidence, dental pain, and OR referrals compared with baseline rates.[43] CDM may hold strong promise to curtail caries activity and complement dental repair when needed, while also reducing disease progression and caries recurrence.[43,45]

PART 3: EMERGENCY DEPARTMENT DISCHARGES FOR DENTAL CONDITIONS AMONG CHILDREN AGED 0 TO 20 YEARS FROM 2010 TO 2014

The use of emergency departments (ED) for routine care or treatment of preventable dental conditions is an escalating public health concern for health care policymakers and providers across the United States.[46–49] Like the OR, the ED is a place where the costs of care delivery are very high. However, in the ED, the dental care received is usually only palliative.[50] More than 90% of DOHRC visits to the ED result in no dental procedures received,[51] and only result in prescriptions for acute management of pain and infection. Given the excessive cost and poor outcomes of treatment of DOHRC in the ED, multiple studies have addressed the reasons for these visits, and how to avoid them.[1,46,47,49,52] However, with few exceptions,[48] there has been no systematic research done on ED use among pediatric patients.

Pediatric ED visits for dental conditions are of particular interest to clinicians, researchers, and policymakers because they should be more avoidable than adult visits. As stated earlier, dental care and insurance coverage are more widely available to children through the EPSDT benefit of Medicaid[53] and school-based and community-based programs.[54,55] However, even with the availability of these benefits, there remain significant barriers to achieving optimal oral health, and access to oral health care, among children.[2,12,13] These barriers are often related to the cost of dental care.[1,2] Here, trends in pediatric ED discharges for nontraumatic dental conditions in the United States from 2010 to 2014 are described.

Methods

The data used in this descriptive analysis came from the National Emergency Department Sample (NEDS) databases 2010 to 2014.[56] NEDS provides estimates of all ED visits in the United States. All statistics were weighted as recommended by the Healthcare Cost and Utilization Project (HCUP).[57] Rates per 100,000 of population were calculated using census population estimates.[58]

As discussed earlier, DOHRC were defined as ICD-9-CM diagnosis codes 520.0 through 529.9. Variables indicating preventability and severity of DOHRC were created using a schema that classifies ICD-9-CM dental diagnosis codes based on the severity of the conditions and the likelihood that the conditions were preventable through normal dental care.[47] Comorbidities were classified using the enhanced Elixhauser classification scheme.[59] Additional variables used in this analysis include age (categorized using EPSDT categories[53]), gender, median household income of the patient's zip code, and the expected payer of costs. The race and ethnicity of patients are not available in the NEDS data.

Results

In 2011, there were 350 ED discharges for DOHRC for every 100,000 children aged 20 and younger (**Table 3**). By 2013, that rate had decreased slightly to 331. Slightly less than half (45.9% in 2013) of ED visits for DOHRC were likely preventable. More than 60% of all DOHRC conditions diagnosed in the ED were considered low severity and did not need urgent care. Consistently over time, DOHRC discharges made up about 1% of all pediatric ED discharges. In contrast, only about 13% of DOHRC discharges occur among those less than 21 years old, whereas more than 25% of medical discharges occur among those less than 21 years old.

Inflation-adjusted charges for DOHRC ED discharges increased from $175 million dollars annually in 2011 to $207 million in 2014, even as the number of pediatric DOHRC ED discharges decreased (**Fig. 4**). More than half of all charges for DOHRC ED discharges are paid for by Medicaid and that proportion has increased over time, reaching 63% and charges totaling $125 million dollars in 2014. About 20% of all charges for DOHRC are paid by private insurance plans or are out-of-pocket payments by uninsured patients. The proportion paid by patients has decreased over

Table 3

Counts and rates of emergency department discharges for dental/oral health–related conditions among children aged 0 to 20 years using National Emergency Department Databases

	2011					2012				
	Number of Discharges	SE	Rate of Discharges per 100,000 Persons	% of all Discharges Caused by DOHRC	% of Total Discharges	Number of Discharges	SE	Rate of Discharges per 100,000 Persons	% of all Discharges Caused by DOHRC	% of Total Discharges
Discharges										
Total ED Discharges	31,297,975	984,303	35,793.35	—	28.1	32,076,059	1,097,774	36,847.80	—	28.8
DOHRC Discharges	306,419	9636	350.43	1.0	12.0	301,264	10,747	346.08	0.9	14.1
DOHRC by Preventability										
Unlikely to be Preventable	14,112	637	16.14	4.6	—	15,190	739	17.45	5.0	—
Possibly Preventable	149,377	4824	170.83	48.7	—	147,656	5471	169.62	49.0	—
Likely Preventable	142,931	5181	163.46	46.6	—	138,417	5292	159.01	45.9	—
DOHRC by Severity										
Low Severity	189,323	5567	216.52	62.4	—	184,953	6413	212.47	61.4	—
Medium Severity	113,718	5157	130.05	37.5	—	112,748	5165	129.52	37.4	—
High Severity	463	50	0.53	0.2	—	493	58	0.57	0.2	—

	2013					2014				
	Number of Discharges	SE	Rate of Discharges per 100,000 Persons	% of all Discharges Caused by DOHRC	% of Total Discharges	Number of Discharges	SE	Rate of Discharges per 100,000 Persons	% of all Discharges Caused by DOHRC	% of Total Discharges
Discharges										
Total ED Discharges	30,667,968	1,252,788	35,357.93	—	27.5	30,302,072	1,030,000	34,999.95	—	26.5
DOHRC Discharges	280,409	11,220	323.29	0.9	13.4	287,335	9913	331.88	0.9	12.9
DOHRC by Preventability										
Unlikely to be Preventable	13,664	722	15.75	4.9	—	16,265	811	18.79	5.7	—
Possibly Preventable	135,874	5301	156.65	48.5	—	139,061	4802	160.62	48.4	—
Likely Preventable	130,871	5117	150.89	46.7	—	132,010	4996	152.48	45.9	—
DOHRC by Severity										
Low Severity	175,273	7193	202.08	63.1	—	177,474	5851	204.99	61.8	—
Medium Severity	101,971	4589	117.57	36.7	—	106,460	4653	122.97	37.1	—
High Severity	369	53	0.43	0.1	—	356	47	0.41	0.1	—

Note: DOHRCs are defined as diagnoses of ICD-9-CM codes 520.0 through 529.9. Weighted national estimates from HCUP National (Nationwide) NEDS, 2011 to 2013, Agency for Healthcare Research and Quality (AHRQ) for patients aged 0 to 20 years. Rates per 100,000 calculated using census information from Census Current Population Estimates. Preventability and severity calculated by schema in Shortridge and Moore[47] (2010).
Data from HCUP Nationwide Emergency Department Sample (NEDS). Healthcare Cost and Utilization Project (HCUP). Agency for Healthcare Research and Quality. 2011–2014. Available at: http://www.hcup-us.ahrq.gov/nedsoverview.jsp. Accessed April 5, 2017.

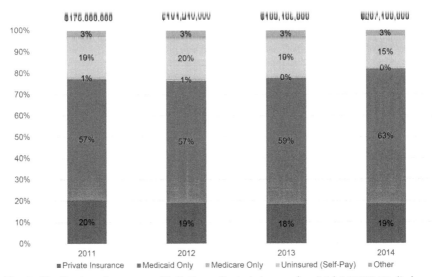

Fig. 4. Distribution of payers and inflation adjusted charges for child DOHRC ED discharges 2011 to 2014. (*Data from* HCUP Nationwide Emergency Department Sample (NEDS). Healthcare Cost and Utilization Project (HCUP). Agency for Healthcare Research and Quality. 2011–2014. Available at: http://www.hcup-us.ahrq.gov/nedsoverview.jsp. Accessed April 5, 2017.)

time, likely because of the expansion of Medicaid coverage through the Affordable Care Act.

Patients aged 19 to 20 years have by far the highest rates of ED visits for DOHRC conditions, compared with other pediatric age groups (**Fig. 5**). This rate is likely an issue of access to dental care and insurance because dental insurance plans are

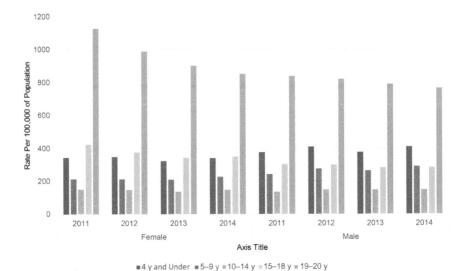

Fig. 5. Gender and age distribution of child DOHRC ED discharges 2011 to 2014. (*Data from* HCUP Nationwide Emergency Department Sample (NEDS). Healthcare Cost and Utilization Project (HCUP). Agency for Healthcare Research and Quality. 2011–2014. Available at: http://www.hcup-us.ahrq.gov/nedsoverview.jsp. Accessed April 5, 2017.)

not required to cover those more than 18 years of age on their parents plans and they are unlikely to have jobs that offer dental insurance.[60] In other age groups, rates of DOHRC visits decline from ages 0 to 14 years, before increasing again at age 15 years. Boys have higher rates of DOHRC ED visits than girls for children less than 9 years old, but girls have substantially higher rates from ages 15 to 20 years.

Pediatric ED discharges for DOHRC are disproportionately concentrated among those who live in impoverished areas (**Fig. 6**). DOHRC are proportionately more likely to occur among those living in the poorest (lowest quartile of median household income) zip codes compared with ED discharges for all reasons.

More than 94% of all pediatric patients discharged with a DOHRC had no Elixhauser comorbidities, 5.5% had 1, and only half of 1% had 2 or more in 2014 (**Table 4**). In comparison, 87% of patients seen in the ED for any reason had no comorbidities, 12% had 1, and 1% had 2 or more. About 3.5% of patients discharged with a DOHRC had a chronic pulmonary disease, whereas about 0.5% had a codiagnosis of depression, hypertension, fluid or electrolyte conditions, or other neurologic disorder.

Discussion

National trends in pediatric ED discharges for DOHRC from 2010 to 2014 are described here. Dental conditions make up a small, but persistent, portion of ED discharges among patients less than 21 old. The dental conditions most commonly seen in the ED for pediatric patients are preventable and of low severity. The costs of these discharges continue to increase over time. The typical pediatric patient who visits the ED for a DOHRC is a poor girl between the ages of 15 and 20 years, who is otherwise healthy.

It is probable that pediatric patients visit the ED for routine and preventable dental conditions most often because of the excessive cost of dental care or dental insurances. Expanding existing benefits, such as increasing Medicaid coverage or allowing children to stay on their caregivers' dental insurance plans until age 26 years (as they can in medical insurance), are likely the best long-term solutions for this public health problem.

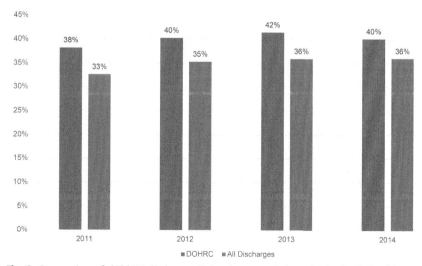

Fig. 6. Proportion of child ED discharges living in poorest zip codes in the United States 2011 to 2013. (*Data from* HCUP Nationwide Emergency Department Sample (NEDS). Healthcare Cost and Utilization Project (HCUP). Agency for Healthcare Research and Quality. 2011–2014. Available at: http://www.hcup-us.ahrq.gov/nedsoverview.jsp. Accessed April 5, 2017.)

Table 4
Counts and rates of Elixhauser comorbidity diagnoses for emergency department discharges for dental/oral health related conditions among children aged 0 to 20 years using the Nationwide Emergency Department Sample

	DOHRC Discharges											
	2011			2012			2013			2014		
Comorbidities	Number of Discharges	Rate per 100,000 Persons	% of Discharges	Number of Discharges	Rate per 100,000 Persons	% of Discharges	Number of Discharges	Rate per 100,000 Persons	% of Discharges	Number of Discharges	Rate per 100,000 Persons	% of Discharges
Counts												
0	289,902	331.54	94.6	284,865	327.24	94.6	263,723	304.05	94.0	270,058	311.93	94.0
1	15,285	17.48	5.0	15,043	17.28	5.0	15,444	17.81	5.5	15,972	18.45	5.6
2+	1232	1.41	0.4	1356	1.56	0.5	1243	1.43	0.4	1305	1.51	0.5
Conditions												
Chronic Pulmonary Disease	10,090	11.54	3.3	9436	10.84	3.1	9850	11.36	3.5	10,601	12.24	3.7
Depression	1461	1.67	0.5	1355	1.56	0.4	1511	1.74	0.5	1263	1.46	0.4
Hypertension, Uncomplicated	1074	1.23	0.4	927	1.06	0.3	837	0.96	0.3	1029	1.19	0.4
Fluid and Electrolyte	973	1.11	0.3	1177	1.35	0.4	996	1.15	0.4	905	1.05	0.3
Other Neurologic Disorders	816	0.93	0.3	939	1.08	0.3	954	1.10	0.3	895	1.03	0.3

All ED Discharges

Comorbidities	2011			2012			2013			2014		
	Number of Discharges	Rate per 100,000 Persons	% of Discharges	Number of Discharges	Rate per 100,000 Persons	% of Discharges	Number of Discharges	Rate per 100,000 Persons	% of Discharges	Number of Discharges	Rate per 100,000 Persons	% of Discharges
Counts												
0	27,283,807	31,202.62	87.2	28,061,872	32,236.45	87.5	26,747,477	30,837.89	87.2	26,287,613	30,363.11	86.8
1	3,691,245	4221.42	11.8	3,682,019	4229.77	11.5	3,581,805	4129.56	11.7	3,653,408	4219.81	12.1
2+	322,923	369.30	1.0	332,168	381.58	1.0	338,686	390.48	1.1	361,051	417.03	1.2
Conditions												
Chronic Pulmonary Disease	2,300,625	2631.07	7.4	2,286,397	2626.53	7.1	2,216,104	2555.01	7.2	2,265,779	2617.05	7.5
Other Neurologic Disorders	399,055	456.37	1.3	393,516	452.06	1.2	384,661	443.49	1.3	397,036	458.59	1.3
Fluid and Electrolyte	412,265	471.48	1.3	410,665	471.76	1.3	400,261	461.47	1.3	369,745	427.07	1.2
Depression	282,660	323.19	0.9	304,519	349.82	0.9	308,153	355.28	1.0	347,700	401.61	1.1
Drug Abuse	173,452	198.41	0.6	176,914	203.23	0.6	180,996	208.68	0.6	189,693	219.10	0.6

Note: DOHRCs are defined as diagnoses of ICD-9-CM codes 520.0 through 529.9. Estimates from NEDS, 2010 to 2014, AHRQ. Elixhauser comorbidities are coded using the AHRQ ICD-9 coding algorithm: https://www.hcup-us.ahrq.gov/toolssoftware/comorbidity/comorbidity.jsp.
Data from HCUP Nationwide Emergency Department Sample (NEDS). Healthcare Cost and Utilization Project (HCUP). Agency for Healthcare Research and Quality. 2011–2014. Available at: http://www.hcup-us.ahrq.gov/nedsoverview.jsp. Accessed April 5, 2017.

SUMMARY

This article describes the interaction between state-level factors and access to dental care for the pediatric Medicaid population. It shows that there is a complicated relationship between Medicaid reimbursement rates, rates of dentist participation in Medicaid, dentist density in the community, patient age, and access to care, including prevention, diagnostic, and treatment services. It also discusses the treatment of DOHRC in the OR, especially among children with special health care needs. It includes analyses showing that most patients treated for DOHRC under GA in the OR could have been treated in less costly settings. In addition, it examines ED visits by pediatric patients for DOHRC. Our results again showed high rates of visits for preventable, nonurgent conditions.

Early access to dental care in conjunction with connecting Medicaid-eligible children with providers is one of the best ways to ensure the provision of the correct prevention and treatment services. Early identification, prevention, and intervention are also crucial to prevent the costly treatment of dental conditions in hospital ORs and EDs. It is clear from the findings presented in this article that what is needed is not increased spending but redirecting spending toward policies designed to provide proper dental care in proper settings.

Policies designed to improve oral health access, and care for both the insured (with enhanced coverage through different types of governmental and nongovernmental insurance and targeted referral programs) and uninsured populations, are required to solve the problems identified in this article. It identifies how increasing reimbursement rates may increase access to care in some states. Dental care coordination is another approach that has shown promising results, including significantly higher dental care use.[61] Solutions will also require active engagement with community-based programs such as Women, Infants, and Children's Supplemental Food Program (WIC) and Head Start, which reach high-risk, low-income children less than 5 years of age and can serve as vehicles for oral health anticipatory guidance while providing early access to dental care.[20]

REFERENCES

1. Vujicic M, Buchmueller T, Klein R. Dental care presents the highest level of financial barriers, compared to other types of health care services. Health Aff (Millwood) 2016;35(12):2176–82.
2. Edelstein BL, Chinn CH. Update on disparities in oral health and access to dental care for America's children. Acad Pediatr 2009;9(6):415–9.
3. Berwick DM, Nolan TW, Whittington J. The triple aim: care, health, and cost. Health Aff (Millwood) 2008;27(3):759–69.
4. Keehan SP, Stone DA, Poisal JA, et al. National health expenditure projections, 2016-25: price increases, aging push sector to 20 percent of economy. Health Aff (Millwood) 2017;36(3):553–63.
5. Dye BA, Thornton-Evans G, Li X, et al. Dental caries and sealant prevalence in children and adolescents in the United States, 2011–2012. NCHS data brief, no 191. Hyattsville (MD): National Center for Health Statistics; 2015.
6. Dieleman JL, Baral R, Birger M, et al. US spending on personal health care and public health, 1996-2013. JAMA 2016;316(24):2627–46.
7. Oral Health in America: a report of the surgeon general. J Calif Dent Assoc 2000; 28(9):685–95.
8. Rosenbaum S. When old is new: Medicaid's EPSDT benefit at fifty, and the future of child health policy. Millbank Q 2016;94(4):716–9.

9. Hom JM, Lee JY, Silverman J, et al. State Medicaid early and periodic screening, diagnosis, and treatment guidelines: adherence to professionally recommended best oral health practices. J Am Dent Assoc 2013;144(3):297–305.

10. Chalmers N, Compton R. Children's access to dental care affected by reimbursement rates, dentist density, and dentist participation in Medicaid. Am J Public Health 2017;107(10):1612–4.

11. Beazoglou T, Douglass J, Myne-Joslin V, et al. Impact of fee increases on dental utilization rates for children living in Connecticut and enrolled in Medicaid. J Am Dent Assoc 2015;146(1):52–60.

12. Buchmueller TC, Orzol S, Shore-Sheppard LD. The effect of Medicaid payment rates on access to dental care among children. Cambridge (MA): National Bureau of Economic Research; 2013.

13. Decker SL. Medicaid payment levels to dentists and access to dental care among children and adolescents. JAMA 2011;306(2):187–93.

14. Nasseh K, Vujicic M. The impact of Medicaid reform on children's dental care utilization in Connecticut, Maryland, and Texas. Health Serv Res 2015;50(4):1236–49.

15. Nasseh K, Vujicic M, Yarbrough C. A ten-year, state-by-state, analysis of Medicaid fee-for-service reimbursement rates for dental care services. Benefits 2014;20:21.

16. American Dental Association HPI. The oral health care system: a state-by-state analysis. 2015. Available at: http://www.ada.org/~/media/ADA/Science%20and%20Research/HPI/OralHealthCare-StateFacts/Oral-Health-Care-System-Full-Report.pdf. Accessed January 20, 2017.

17. Health Policy Institute. Oral health and well-being in the United States. 2016. Available at: http://www.ada.org/en/science-research/health-policy-institute/oral-health-and-well-being.

18. Bernardo R. 2017's States with the best & worst dental health. 2017. Available at: https://wallethub.com/edu/states-with-best-worst-dental-health/31498/#methodology. Accessed February 24, 2017.

19. Texas Health and Human Services. First Dental Home (FDH). 2017. Available at: https://www.dshs.texas.gov/dental/FDH.shtm. Accessed April 26, 2017.

20. Lee JY. Community programs and oral health. 2nd edition. Hoboken (NJ): Early Childhood Oral Health; 2015. p. 245–57.

21. Wadhawan S, Kumar JV, Badner VM, et al. Early childhood caries-related visits to hospitals for ambulatory surgery in New York State. J Public Health Dent 2003;63(1):47–51.

22. Iwasaki M, Sato M, Yoshihara A, et al. Effects of periodontal diseases on diabetes-related medical expenditure. Curr Oral Health Rep 2016;3(1):7–13.

23. Guideline on use of anesthesia personnel in the administration of office-based deep sedation/general anesthesia to the pediatric dental patient. Pediatr Dent 2016;38(6):246–9.

24. Bruen BK, Steinmetz E, Bysshe T, et al. Potentially preventable dental care in operating rooms for children enrolled in Medicaid. J Am Dent Assoc 2016;147(9):702–8.

25. Chi DL, Momany ET, Neff J, et al. Impact of chronic condition status and severity on dental treatment under general anesthesia for Medicaid-enrolled children in Iowa state. Paediatr Anaesth 2010;20(9):856–65.

26. Lalwani K, Kitchin J, Lax P. Office-based dental rehabilitation in children with special healthcare needs using a pediatric sedation service model. J Oral Maxillofac Surg 2007;65(3):427–33.

27. Griffin SO, Gooch BF, Beltran E, et al. Dental services, costs, and factors associated with hospitalization for Medicaid-eligible children, Louisiana 1996-97. J Public Health Dent 2000;60(1):21–7.

20. Churchill SS, Williams JJ, Villareale NL. Characteristics of publicly insured children with high dental expenses. J Public Health Dent 2007;67(4):199–207.

29. Kanellis MJ, Damiano PC, Momany ET. Medicaid costs associated with the hospitalization of young children for restorative dental treatment under general anesthesia. J Public Health Dent 2000;60(1):28–32.

30. Samnaliev M, Wijeratne R, Kwon EG, et al. Cost-effectiveness of a disease management program for early childhood caries. J Public Health Dent 2015;75(1):24–33.

31. Acs G, Shulman R, Ng MW, et al. The effect of dental rehabilitation on the body weight of children with early childhood caries. Pediatr Dent 1999;21(2):109–13.

32. Cantekin K, Yildirim MD, Cantekin I. Assessing change in quality of life and dental anxiety in young children following dental rehabilitation under general anesthesia. Pediatr Dent 2014;36(1):12E–7E.

33. Bolan M, Cardoso M, Galato G, et al. Overdenture for total rehabilitation in a child with early childhood caries. Pediatr Dent 2012;34(2):148–9.

34. Berkowitz RJ, Amante A, Kopycka-Kedzierawski DT, et al. Dental caries recurrence following clinical treatment for severe early childhood caries. Pediatr Dent 2011;33(7):510–4.

35. Almeida AG, Roseman MM, Sheff M, et al. Future caries susceptibility in children with early childhood caries following treatment under general anesthesia. Pediatr Dent 2000;22(4):302–6.

36. Eidelman E, Faibis S, Peretz B. A comparison of restorations for children with early childhood caries treated under general anesthesia or conscious sedation. Pediatr Dent 2000;22(1):33–7.

37. Graves CE, Berkowitz RJ, Proskin HM, et al. Clinical outcomes for early childhood caries: influence of aggressive dental surgery. J Dent Child (Chic) 2004;71(2): 114–7.

38. Litsas G. Effect of full mouth rehabilitation on the amount of Streptococcus mutans in children with early childhood caries. Eur J Paediatr Dent 2010;11(1):35–8.

39. Li Y, Tanner A. Effect of antimicrobial interventions on the oral microbiota associated with early childhood caries. Pediatr Dent 2015;37(3):226–44.

40. Lin Y-T, Lin Y-TJ. Survey of comprehensive restorative treatment for children under general anesthesia. J Dent Sci 2015;10(3):296–9.

41. Al-Eheideb A, Herman N. Outcomes of dental procedures performed on children under general anesthesia. J Clin Pediatr Dent 2004;27(2):181–3.

42. Feudtner C, Feinstein JA, Zhong W, et al. Pediatric complex chronic conditions classification system version 2: updated for ICD-10 and complex medical technology dependence and transplantation. BMC Pediatr 2014;14:199.

43. Edelstein BL, Ng MW. Chronic disease management strategies of early childhood caries: support from the medical and dental literature. Pediatr Dent 2015;37(3):281–7.

44. Ng MW, Fida Z. Early childhood caries disease prevention and management. 2nd edition. Hoboken (NJ): Early Childhood Oral Health; 2015. p. 47–66.

45. Ng MW, Ramos-Gomez F, Lieberman M, et al. Disease management of early childhood caries: ECC collaborative project. Int J Dent 2014;2014:327801.

46. Wall T, Vujicic M. Emergency department use for dental conditions continues to increase. Chicago (IL): Health Policy Institute Research Brief; 2015. Available at: http://www.ada.org/~/media/ADA/Science%20and%20Research/HPI/Files/HPI-Brief_0415_2.ashx.

47. Shortridge EF, Moore JR. Use of emergency departments for conditions related to poor oral health care. Bethesda (MD): NORC Walsh Center for Rural Health Analysis; 2010.

48. Dorfman DH, Kastner B, Vinci RJ. Dental concerns unrelated to trauma in the pediatric emergency department: barriers to care. Arch Pediatr Adolesc Med 2001; 155(6):699–703.

49. Chalmers N, Grover J, Compton R. After Medicaid expansion in Kentucky, use of hospital emergency departments for dental conditions increased. Health Aff 2016;35(12):2268–76.

50. Cohen LA, Bonito AJ, Eicheldinger C, et al. Comparison of patient visits to emergency departments, physician offices, and dental offices for dental problems and injuries. J Public Health Dent 2011;71(1):13–22.

51. McCormick AP, Abubaker AO, Laskin DM, et al. Reducing the burden of dental patients on the busy hospital emergency department. J Oral Maxillofac Surg 2013;71(3):475–8.

52. Quinonez C, Gibson D, Jokovic A, et al. Emergency department visits for dental care of nontraumatic origin. Community Dent Oral Epidemiol 2009;37(4):366–71.

53. Centers for Medicare & Medicaid Services. Early and periodic screening, diagnostic, and treatment. 2017. Available at: https://www.medicaid.gov/medicaid/benefits/epsdt/index.html. Accessed April 19, 2017.

54. Gooch BF, Griffin SO, Gray SK, et al. Preventing dental caries through school-based sealant programs. J Am Dent Assoc 2009;140(11):1356–65.

55. Mandal M, Edelstein BL, Ma S, et al. Changes in state policies related to oral health in the United States, 2002-2009. J Public Health Dent 2014;74(4):266–75.

56. (HCUP) Healthcare Cost and Utilization Project. NEDS overview. 2017. Available at: www.hcup-us.ahrq.gov/nedsoverview.jsp. Accessed April 19, 2017.

57. Houchens RRD, Elixhauser A. Final report on calculating national inpatient sample (NIS) variances for data years 2012 and later. Rockville (MD): U.S. Agency for Healthcare Research and Quality; 2015.

58. United States Census Bureau. National population by characteristics tables: 2010-2016. Available at: https://www.census.gov/data/tables/2016/demo/popest/nation-detail.html. Accessed April 19, 2017.

59. Quan H, Sundararajan V, Halfon P, et al. Coding algorithms for defining comorbidities in ICD-9- CM and ICD-10 administrative data. Med Care 2005;43(11):1130–9.

60. Center for Consumer Information & Insurance Oversight. Information on Essential Health Benefits (EHB) Benchmark Plans. Available at: https://www.cms.gov/cciio/resources/data-resources/ehb.html. Accessed April 20, 2017.

61. Binkley CJ, Garrett B, Johnson KW. Increasing dental care utilization by Medicaid-eligible children: a dental care coordinator intervention. J Public Health Dent 2010;70(1):76–84.

Innovative Models of Dental Care Delivery and Coverage

Patient-Centric Dental Benefits Based on Digital Oral Health Risk Assessment

John Martin, DDS[a], Shannon Mills, DDS[b], Mary E. Foley, MPH, RDH[c],*

KEYWORDS

- Dental care • Dental benefits • Preventive • Risk-based care
- Risk-assessment technology • Cloud-based technology • Patient-centered care
- Evidence-based

KEY POINTS

- The purpose of innovative models is to align the interests and activities of all stakeholders to provide quality oral health care.
- Quality oral health care is defined and measured by clinical and patient-centric outcomes.
- The models' primary focus of oral health care is to sustain wellness by prevention in contrast to disease-necessitated repair.
- A key element is digital risk and severity assessment, which allow for objective precise measurement of oral health status and outcomes.
- Risk assessment expands on traditional diagnosis and repair by including risk as a modifier of treatment and as a determinant of preventive services.

DENTAL BENEFITS, EVIDENCE-BASED DENTISTRY, AND HEALTH CARE QUALITY

According to data from the Centers for Medicare and Medicaid Services, an estimated $117.5 billion or $366 per person was spent on dental services in 2015 by individuals, private insurers, and government payers.[1] There is, however, little objective evidence

Disclosure Statement: Drs J. Martin and S. Mills have a financial interest in the commercial product(s) or service(s) discussed in this article. M.E. Foley, as a representative of the Medicaid Medicare CHIP Services Dental Association, has a financial affiliation with the PreViser Corporation.

[a] PreViser Corporation, 2521 Carnegie Drive, State College, PA 16803, USA; [b] PreViser Corporation, 2 Delta Drive, Suite 302, Concord, NH 03302-2002, USA; [c] Medicaid, Medicare, CHIP Services Dental Association, 4411 Connecticut Avenue NorthWest, Suite 401, Washington, DC 20008, USA
* Corresponding author.
E-mail address: Mfoley@medicaiddental.org

to show that these expenditures resulted in improvements in the oral health of individuals or populations receiving these dental services.[2]

Innovative models of dental care delivery and coverage are being developed to align the interests and activities of patients, purchasers, payers, and providers to provide quality oral health care as defined by the Institute of Medicine, which the authors paraphrase as *"the degree to which (oral) health services increase the likelihood of a patient's desired outcome and is consistent with current professional knowledge."*[3] These models expand on the traditional disease, diagnosis, and repair approach by emphasizing the value of risk prediction and prevention. Hence, the models' primary focus of dental care is to sustain wellness by prevention in contrast to disease-necessitated repair.

Innovative models of dental care delivery and coverage are being developed as a response to the need for evidence-based practice models that use dental quality measures to help dental professionals achieve outcomes desired by their patients.[3–5] Traditional dental quality measures have assessed the process of care, such as access, safety, conformity with guidelines, and technical standards of care, and patient satisfaction with the care experience. Outcomes follow the process of care. Accordingly, the new models incorporate outcomes composed of clinical outcomes and outcomes from the patient's perspective, such as quality-of-life measures and patient-reported outcomes.

The process of dental care, illustrated in **Fig. 1**, ends with outcomes, which are the foundational measure of dental care quality.[3,6–8] The value proposition for oral health services can be defined as outcomes relative to costs.[6] Although outcomes themselves have no associated cost, cost affects outcomes by its influence on access to care, the selection and delivery of services, and patient satisfaction with the care experience. Patient satisfaction can also exert a powerful force on outcomes and quality. Elements affecting patient satisfaction with care include the physical environment, dentist-patient-staff interactions, and the patient's perceived value of objective treatment outcomes.[9] Therefore, cost reduction or increase without consideration of outcomes may adversely affect the value proposition of health care services.

To achieve the best outcomes, new oral health care models will require the use of information technology that aligns the interests of purchasers, patients, third-party

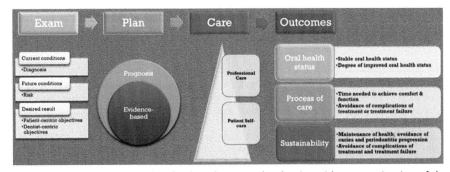

Fig. 1. Outcomes are the results of a dental process that begins with an examination of the patient, development of a treatment plan, and care. The examination includes an assessment of current conditions, future conditions, and desired results of care. Evidence-based and prognostic information is used along with the examination assessment to plan treatment. The results of care include outcomes about oral health status, the care process, and status during a follow-on period.

payers, and providers. Using objective measures of disease severity and risk, third-party payers can create plan designs that encourage provider performance congruent with recommended best clinical practices. These systems must also provide accessible resources to help patients make educated health care decisions.

Among the challenges the profession faces in transitioning from procedure-based payment to a system that rewards better outcomes is that third-party payers do not typically require submission of diagnostic codes or other information describing the clinical condition of the patient. The available information is a record of financial transactions between the provider and the payer for services rendered resulting in an estimate of value, cost-benefit, and quality based on claims data. Without objective descriptions of clinical findings or a diagnosis, these estimates provide, at best, an imprecise surrogate measure for the patient's true oral health status and outcomes of care. The lack of objective clinical findings limits the capacity to analyze the effects of oral health care and impedes the development of ways to improve outcomes and value-based reimbursement systems.[5,6,8]

Several investigators have identified the need for information systems that use objective clinical information provided by the patient or entered by the provider at chairside to measure an individual's current oral health status and estimate risk for future disease.[7,10–12] A standardized set of oral health risk and disease severity scores can provide clinical decision support for diagnosis and treatment planning by the provider; focused engagement of patients to motivate behavioral change; and evidence-based preventive care benefit determinations from third-party payers based on individual risk for oral disease.

Current evidence-based guidelines from both the American Dental Association and the American Association of Pediatric Dentistry base both the intensity and the frequency for preventive services on the individual patient's risk for dental caries. These guidelines recommend that children at greater risk for dental caries receive up to 4 fluoride treatments per year and that fluoride treatment is most likely beneficial for adults at greater risk as well.[13,14] Caries risk assessment tools that are available to assist clinicians in evidence-based treatment planning include Caries Management by Risk Assessment or CAMBRA,[15] Caries Risk Assessment,[16] and Caries Assessment Test.[14]

Data systems that allow a dental provider to accurately convey objective clinical information about a patient to the dental insurer for automated predetermination of evidence-based benefits and to the patient for oral health counseling can be an important step in creating a more patient-centric and evidence-based dental care model. The American Dental Association Standards Committee for Dental Informatics has anticipated the need for voluntary consensus in the development of these technologies and recently published a standard describing the essential characteristics of digital oral health risk assessment resources.[17]

A CLOUD-BASED SYSTEM FOR A RISK-BASED MODEL OF DENTAL BENEFITS AND CARE

In 2010, a regional dental insurance carrier operating in Maine, New Hampshire, and Vermont (Northeast Delta Dental, Concord, NH, USA) began a novel collaboration with a health care technology company specializing in digital oral health risk and disease severity measurement (PreViser Corporation, Concord, NH, USA and Mount Vernon, Washington, USA) to pilot a patient-centric dental plan design whereby patients would have access to evidence-based benefits matched to their individual needs based on submission of a standardized assessment of disease severity and risk. The plan design became known as Health through Oral Wellness or HOW.

PreViser had previously developed a clinical risk assessment measure called the Oral Health Information Suite or OHIS, which provides scientifically validated measures for periodontal disease risk, severity, and stability,[18–20] which was in use by dentists in the United States, the United Kingdom, and Japan. Other measures of OHIS that supported the initiative included a caries risk assessment score adapted from the CAMBRA analogue risk assessment tool,[15] a restorative needs score, and an oral cancer risk score.

Embedded algorithms in PreViser's cloud computing service use standardized information about the patient to create objective and repeatable measures describing the patient's current oral health status and risk for future disease. Oral Health Risk and Severity Reports generated by the OHIS and downloaded at chairside, use color-coded numerical scores to help the patient understand their current oral health status and risk for future disease along with evidence-based preventive care and treatment recommendations.

Aggregated risk and severity data from the OHIS can also be used to create population oral health profiles and potentially to define clinically derived outcome measures. When compared with claims data, these clinical measures can identify gaps in care that can be addressed through patient-centric and evidence-based plan designs, patient engagement, provider education, and value-based reimbursement to achieve better clinical outcomes.

In a 2-year pilot program with 2 employer groups, the dental insurer developed a plan design that provided suites of enhanced preventive dental benefits based on evidence-based guidelines for preventive care from dental professional organizations, including the American Dental Association, the American Academy of Pediatric Dentistry, and the American Academy of Periodontology. Initially, both analogue and PreViser digital risk assessments were accepted by the insurer for making benefit determinations. It became soon apparent, however, that analogue assessments were administratively unscalable. To operationalize an evidence-based plan design across the company's book of business, a single, standardized, digital risk assessment tool set became an essential requirement.

USE OF AN INFORMATION SYSTEM TO IMPROVE HEALTH CARE QUALITY

To operationalize the HOW program, PreViser and Northeast Delta Dental began a collaboration to build a secure cloud-based platform that came to be called the Population Oral Health Manager (POHM). The features of the POHM, shown diagrammatically in **Fig. 2**, include a HIPAA compliant cloud computing services and data storage hub that contains encrypted OHIS-generated patient data. These data are then accessible through a data hub that resides behind the dental insurer firewall using a decryption key known only to the patient's provider, dental insurer, or other HIPAA authorized user.

The data hub can access or share data with the provider's electronic health record and the dental insurer's claims payment system for automated benefit determination. The POHM Platform also includes a digital messaging center that provides automated messaging to engage patients based on user-defined characteristics.

In addition to scores, the reports provide actionable information regarding evidence-based preventive care or treatment recommendations to restore health and/or prevent disease. The risk and severity scores can be correlated with current diagnostic criteria to provide diagnostic decision support for the provider.

By transmitting oral health data scores directly to the patient's dental insurer to automatically trigger a predetermination of the evidence-based benefits, the need for administrative or consultant review is avoided, making the transaction virtually

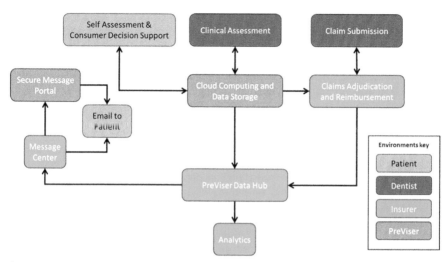

Fig. 2. Core components of the POHM include cloud computing services, data storage hub, and message center. Embedded algorithms in the cloud computing service return a description of the patient's current oral health status and risk for future disease. An insurer using information in the data storage hub adjudicates claims, analyzes care, and sends health care messages of particular importance to a specific patient.

instantaneous, which results in savings in administrative costs for both the benefit plan and the provider.

In contrast to plan designs that provide additional cleanings or other benefits based on medical diagnoses such as diabetes or pregnancy, risk-based benefit programs like HOW focus on primary prevention of oral disease and do not require the patient to be diagnosed with a systemic comorbidity to obtain evidence-based dental benefits.

The HOW plan was made available to all of the dental insurer's employer groups in January 2015, and by June 2017, more than 99% of the insurer's employer groups adopted the new plan design. The program could not succeed without adequate clinician participation. Fortunately, provider acceptance has exceeded expectations, with more than 86% of plan participating and nonparticipating licensed dentists in the insurer's coverage area of Maine, New Hampshire, and Vermont accepting free licenses to use the OHIS clinical tool. These dentists have submitted more than 76,000 risk assessments as of June 2017. Although it is too early at this time to assess the impact of the new plan design on outcomes or quality measures, a nonscientific survey of dentists found high levels of user satisfaction with the program. There has been no increase in premium costs or administrative expense for employers attributable to the program.

WHY SCORES MATTER

Numerical scores are integral to evidence-based and patient-centric care and benefit models. PreViser's information system provides objective and repeatable measures describing a patient's oral health status and its change over time. Some elements of the scoring system have been scientifically validated, whereas others are still based predominantly on expert opinion. Standardized assessment measures, however, provide the only way to establish a basis for quality assessment, economic analysis, and patient-centered care.[2,3,6,8,21]

Scores can be used to describe current conditions or to predict the likelihood a condition will occur or worsen in the future (ie, disease risk assessment). In addition to scores that measure a patient's condition over time or describe treatment outcomes, scores that describe the patient's satisfaction with their oral health and treatment received are also important (eg, oral health–related quality of life, patient-reported outcomes). Patient activation measures can be developed to measure a patient's level of understanding of their oral health status and their ability and willingness to participate in self-care activities to improve health outcomes.

Implementation of dental diagnostic codes will be an important advance that will drive improvements in oral health care quality. Objective, clinically based, risk, severity, and stability scores can enhance the accuracy of diagnosis and provide additional granularity to reveal changes in oral health over time within a diagnostic classification. For example, the OHIS periodontal health module describes periodontal status by applying weighted values for pocket depth, supporting bone and bleeding on probing, using a computerized algorithm. A numerical scale from 1 (representing gingival health) to 100 (representing severe periodontitis in all dentate sextants) describes the extent of disease severity within each diagnostic class. For each diagnostic descriptor, other than "health," there are multiple scores for gingivitis, mild periodontitis, moderate periodontitis, and severe periodontitis. Each score accurately and precisely describes a current condition, which means the outcomes of improvement and deterioration are captured with greater granularity than is possible with purely descriptive diagnostic nomenclature or codes.

SUMMARY

The use of digital risk-assessment technology offers a promising new approach for models of dental care and benefits that has value for patients, purchasers, payers, and providers. The dental benefit provider uses risk assessment scores to automatically predetermine evidence-based preventive benefits for patients at greater risk for oral disease. This, in turn, reduces barriers to case acceptance and patient compliance that occur when coverage for evidence-based services is denied based on age or frequency limitations. Although it is too early in the program to demonstrate improvement in outcomes, purchaser, provider, and patient acceptance has been very favorable with no significant increase in costs to purchasers.

Digital risk and severity assessment allows for more objective and granular measurement of oral health status for individuals and populations than claims data or diagnostic codes alone. Digital risk assessment resources like the OHIS and POHM may help bridge the divide between the current fee-for-service model with payment based primarily on actuarial rather than clinical measures and truly value-based reimbursement models based on achieving objectively measured clinical outcomes.

REFERENCES

1. Available at: https://www.cms.gov/research-statistics-data-and-systems/statistics-trends-and-reports/nationalhealthexpenddata/nationalhealthaccountshistorical.html. Accessed April 14, 2017.
2. Bader JD. Challenges in quality assessment of dental care. J Am Dent Assoc 2009;140:1456–64.
3. Crossing the quality chasm: a new health system for the 21st century. Committee on quality health care in America, Institute of Medicine. Washington, DC: National Academy of Sciences; 2001.
4. American Dental Association, Evidence-based dentistry–Clinical Practice Guidelines; Available at: http://ebd.ada.org/en/evidence/guidelines. Accessed August 14, 2017.

5. American Dental Association, Dental Quality Alliance; DQA measures activities; Available at: http://www.ada.org/en/science-research/dental-quality-alliance/dqa-measure-activities; Accessed August 14, 2017.
6. Porter ME. What is value in health care? N Engl J Med 2010;363:2477–81.
7. Bader JD, Ismail AI. A primer on outcomes in dentistry. J Public Health Dent 1999; 59:131–5.
8. NCQA Essential guide to health care quality. URL: Available at: http://www.ncqa.org/Portals/0/Publications/Resource%20Library/NCQA_Primer_web.pdf?ver= 2007 03 21-112202-000. Accessed April 12, 2016.
9. Lytle RS, Mokwa MP. Evaluating health care quality: the moderating role of outcomes. J Health Care Mark 1992;12:4–14.
10. Porter ME, Teisberg EO. Redefining competition in health care. Harv Bus Rev 2004;82:64–76.
11. Bader JD, Shugars DA. A case for diagnoses. J Am Coll Dent 1997;64:44–6.
12. Enthoven AC, Vorhaus CB. A vision of quality in health care delivery. Health Aff 1997;16:44–57.
13. Available at: http://www.ada.org/en/member-center/oral-health-topics/caries-risk-assessment-and-management. Accessed on August 14, 2017.
14. American Association of Pediatric Dentistry Council on Clinical Affairs; policy on caries risk assessment; 2014 Available at: http://www.aapd.org/media/policies_guidelines/g_cariesriskassessment.pdf. Accessed August 14, 2017.
15. Featherstone JD. The caries balance: the basis for caries management by risk assessment. Oral Health Prev Dent 2004;2(Suppl 1):259–64.
16. American Dental Association Foundation; ADA Caries Risk Assessment Form Completion Instructions; Available at: http://www.adafoundation.org/~/media/ADA_Foundation/GKAS/Files/topics_caries_instructions_GKAS.pdf?la=en. Accessed August 14, 2017.
17. American Dental Association Standards Committee for Dental Informatics: Technical Report 1087-2017–Essential Characteristics of Digital Oral Health Risk Assessment Resources; Available at: http://ebusiness.ada.org/productcatalog/33785/Informatics/ADA1087-2017. Accessed August 14, 2017.
18. Page RC, Krall EA, Martin JA, et al. Validity and accuracy of a risk calculator in predicting periodontal disease. J Am Dent Assoc 2002;133:569–76.
19. Page RC, Martin J, Krall EA, et al. Longitudinal validation of a risk calculator for periodontal disease. J Clin Periodontol 2003;30:819–27.
20. Page RC, Martin JA. Quantification of periodontal risk and disease severity and extent using the Oral Health Information Suite (OHIS). Periodontal Pract Today 2007;4:163–80.
21. Committee on Core Metrics for Better Health at Lower Cost, Institute of Medicine, The National Academies of Sciences, Engineering, and Medicine. Vital Signs: Core Metrics for Health and Health Care Progress. In: Blumenthal D, Malphrus E, McGinnis JM, editors. Washington, DC: The National Academies Press; 2015. Available at: https://www.ncbi.nlm.nih.gov/pubmed/26378329 Accessed January 11, 2018.

A Public Health Perspective on Paying for Dentistry, the Affordable Care Act, and Looking to the Future

Burton L. Edelstein, DDS, MPH[a,b,]*

KEYWORDS

- Triple aim/3-part aim • Value • Iron triangle • Payment innovation
- Dental care financing • Dental public health

KEY POINTS

- US health care financing is moving from volume-to-value as public and private payers seek improved health outcomes at lower cost.
- Conviction that cost, quality, and access present oppositional tradeoffs is being challenged as health care providers are financially incentivized through alternative payment mechanisms to reform health care with a focus on health outcomes rather than health care procedures.
- The Affordable Care Act (ACA) stimulated value-based innovation through a range of federally sponsored demonstrations and incentives.
- Efforts to repeal the ACA evinced a range of conservative approaches, some of which would reduce the numbers of people covered and reduce dental coverage.
- Dental public health philosophies, interventions, and skills are essential to integrating oral health within this complex and dynamic era of health reform.

Disclosure: Dr B.L. Edelstein reports no financial conflicts of interest. With regard to references in this article, he discloses that the MySmileBuddy early childhood caries research he directs is currently sponsored by the federal Center for Medicare & Medicaid Innovation (C1CMS331347) and that he serves as a subcontractor to the Centers for Medicare & Medicaid Services Innovation Accelerator Program Pediatric Oral Health Initiative through the Children's Dental Health Project.

a Population Oral Health, Columbia University College of Dental Medicine, Columbia University Medical Center, 622 West 168th Street, PH7-311, Box 20, New York, NY 10032, USA;
b Children's Dental Health Project, Washington, DC, USA
* Population Oral Health, Columbia University College of Dental Medicine, Columbia University Medical Center, 622 West 168th Street, PH7-311, Box 20, New York, NY 10032.
E-mail address: ble22@columbia.edu

Dent Clin N Am 62 (2018) 327–340
https://doi.org/10.1016/j.cden.2017.12.002
0011-8532/18/© 2017 Elsevier Inc. All rights reserved.

dental.theclinics.com

THE QUEST FOR VALUE IN HEALTH CARE FINANCING

Health care consumers, like all consumers, seek to get what they pay for. This holds true whether the health care consumer is a public health authority, a government, an employer, a union, a purchasing cooperative, an individual, or anything or anyone else charged with distributing scarce resources as effectively and efficiently as possible with the goal of improving and maintaining health.

Securing the most good for each dollar spent is the definition of value. To be successful, therefore, sellers of goods and services must demonstrate, or at least make a claim for, value. Providers of products and services claim value by asserting a value proposition:

> A value proposition is a business or marketing statement that a company uses to summarize why a consumer should buy a product or use a service. This statement convinces a potential consumer that one particular product or service will add more value or better solve a problem than other similar offerings.[1]

What then is dentistry's—in particular, dental public health's—value proposition? What arguments can be put forth to claim that particular clinical or programmatic offerings to oral health enhancement add more value or better solve the problem of poor oral health than competing offerings in dentistry? When comparing clinical care with the range of services available from dental public health authorities, what arguments are available to claim that public health services add more value or better solve oral health problems than clinical care alone? In an environment of ever greater oral health disparities and evermore limited financial resources, what can be expected of consumer and policymaker support for oral health? Will these purchasers elect to prioritize dental care and dental public health spending over competing health and social welfare issues?

This article seeks to place these questions within the larger frameworks of (1) tradeoffs, constraints, and opportunities in dental care financing and delivery and (2) impact of federal policy on dental care financing.

MOVING FROM THE IRON TRIANGLE TO THE 3-PART AIM AND DELIVERY INNOVATION

For all of health care, the traditional value proposition is that doctors, dentists, hospitals and other health care providers know what is best for a person—whether the person is called client, consumer, customer, or patient. They also know what is best for the payer—whether dollars that pay for care originate from individuals, employers, or governments. It is assumed and accepted by both persons and payers that charges levied are inherently appropriate to the quality, quantity, and potential benefit of each health service. Under this paradigm, more health care equates to better health care; more costly health care is more valuable than less costly health care; and health care is regarded as a significant, or even the primary, determinant of health outcomes. This understanding has led to the concept of the iron triangle, in which cost, access, and quality—quality of both care and benefits—function in tension with one another as tradeoffs. Under this conceptualization, desired goals can be accomplished only through compromise. Greater access to care necessitates either higher cost or lesser quality of care or benefits. Lower cost necessitates either lesser access or poorer quality of care or benefits. And greater access either costs more or requires poorer care or skimpier benefits.[2]

Dealing with these tradeoffs was central to the Patient Protection and Affordable Care Act (ACA) of 2010, or Obamacare. The law addressed the cost component of the iron triangle by providing extensive federal financial subsidies to states, employers, and individuals so that more people could be covered by health insurance that ensured comprehensive essential health benefits (EHBs) and assured greater financial access to care. These subsidies included premium assistance, deductible and copayment assistance (albeit legislatively questionable), and enhanced federal support to states that elected to expand their Medicaid offerings. Having made health coverage affordable, the law then sought to promote more efficient and effective care that would enhance value by improving health outcomes at lower costs. Thus the Institute for Healthcare Improvement concept of "triple aim"[3] (known within the federal government as the "3-part aim"[4]) was widely adopted. The triple aim anticipates better individual and population health outcomes at lower cost with enhanced patient or population experience by having health care providers work smarter, not harder—to assess conventional treatments for value that is measured in terms of their contribution to health outcomes—in brief, to transform health care financing from volume-based to value-based.

The ACA flagship creation for reforming the content of health care, including dental care, was the establishment of the federal Center for Medicare & Medicaid Innovation (CMMI) within the Centers for Medicare & Medicaid Services (CMS). CMMI was charged with advancing value-based care over volume-based care by providing grants to states and nonprofit agencies to conduct value demonstrations. CMMI's official mission statement captures this volume-to-value transition:

The CMS Innovation Center fosters healthcare transformation by finding new ways to pay for and deliver care that can lower costs and improve care. The Innovation Center identifies, tests and spreads new ways to pay for and deliver better care and better health at reduced costs through improvement for all Americans.[5]

Value-based initiatives established by the CMMI to reform health care delivery and financing include the Delivery System Reform Incentive Payment (DSRIP) waiver program, the State Innovation Models initiative, the Medicaid Innovation Accelerator Program in collaboration with the National Governors Association,[6] and Health Care Innovation Awards (HCIA) to private nonprofits.[7] Common to each of these programs is the motive to address the iron triangle by demonstrating that better health outcomes are achievable at lower cost, with better population health and patient experience if care systems are redesigned with a focus on efficiency and effectiveness to yield measurable health outcomes.

Consistent with public health–think, many of the endeavors sponsored by these programs address health determinants other than health care, specifically environmental, social, and behavioral health determinants. They feature population health management techniques, including population triage with care tailored to subgroups with differential risk levels. Many demonstrations are grounded in prevention and chronic disease management techniques like the Wagner[8] model of chronic disease management or use new communications technologies, such as telehealth and interoperable electronic health record platforms. Some demonstrations delegate to helping professionals, including health educators, nutritionists, and social workers, as well as lay health workers.

The chair of the federal Medicaid and Children's Health Insurance Program (CHIP) Payment and Access Commission noted in June 2015, "The DSRIP approach, if taken to scale, has the potential to fundamentally change Medicaid's role from financing medical care to driving system change toward value and improved health outcomes."[9] Yet few, if any, DSRIP programs attend specifically to oral health and dental care. New York State's DSRIP Prevention Agenda addresses oral health tangentially by

mandating inclusion of smoking cessation programs across its entire health care system with their salutary oral health implications, especially among low-income populations and beneficiaries with poor mental health. But the Agenda does not reference
oral health specifically.[10]

Among State Innovation Models initiative state grantees, at least 3 of 38 funded
states—Connecticut, Oregon, and Virginia—have incorporated oral health and dental
care into their programs.[11] Reforms by these states and other states using a variety of
other funding sources have been clustered by the Center for Health Care Strategies
into 3 approaches: (1) endeavors to expand the scope of the adult Medicaid dental
benefit or extend Medicaid dental services to new populations, such as pregnant
women and people with diabetes; (2) endeavors to reform dental practice through
scope-of-practice expansions, new workflows, and novel referral networks; and (3)
endeavors to reform statewide delivery systems, such as exploring "coordination between oral and physical health care entities in a value-based payment model."

The federal Center for Medicaid and CHIP Services (CMCS) has capitalized on the
Innovation Accelerator Program approach to tackle the persistent problem of early
childhood caries (ECC) by implementing an oral health initiative entitled, "Children's
Oral Health Initiative Value-Based Payment Technical Support."[12] This program has
compiled a descriptive anthology of 18 ECC programs from across the country that
meet criteria of incorporating disease management strategies, addressing oral health
outcomes, addressing children under age 6 years at risk for or having experience with
ECC, and being amenable to alternative payment arrangements. Referencing these
sources, states were encouraged to compete for technical assistance support from
CMS to implement and evaluate Medicaid oral health innovation programs statewide.
Michigan with a focus on medical-dental integration, New Hampshire with an
approach that targets early intervention through Women, Infants, and Children programs, and the District of Columbia with a proposal to implement pharmacologic disease management with topical fluorides were selected for technical assistance and
coaching that is provided by process and content contractors, including Truven/
IBM, Deloitte, and the Children's Dental Health Project.

CMMI's HCIA program, as of mid-2017, has sponsored 3 oral health–related projects (less than 1.5% of all HCIA funded projects[13]), each of which focuses on a
low-income pediatric population. The first, entitled, "Improving the care and oral
health of American Indian mothers and young children and American Indian people
with diabetes on South Dakota reservations" (the Circle of Smiles program) was
awarded to the Delta Dental of South Dakota from 2012 to 2015. This $3.4 million pro-
gram fielded dental hygienists and "community health representatives" (lay health
workers) in concert with "diabetic program coordinators" among a population of La-
kota Sioux that experiences high rates of caries and diabetes with the goal of reducing
the volume of surgical dental repair in young children to yield a proposed net cost savings to South Dakota Medicaid of $6.2 million dollars. The program notes that savings
are to be generated through "preventive care [that] will help avoid and arrest oral and
dental diseases, repair damage, prevent recurrence, and ultimately, reduce the need
for surgical care."[14] The second round of HCIA funding, from 2014 to 2017, included
2 oral health–related awards. The Altarum Institute, in collaboration with the Michigan
Medicaid program, was awarded $9.4 million for a program entitled, "Reducing the
Burden of Childhood Dental Disease in Michigan," that addressed the oral health
of children and youth under age 18 years by promoting adoption of caries risk
assessment tools by primary care pediatric medical providers; creating a referral linkage systems between medical and dental providers through a health information ex-
change; training medical providers to deliver fluoride varnish and other preventive

strategies; and establishing a statewide dental quality monitoring system using the American Dental Association pediatric oral health starter set.[15] The third HCIA-funded program was awarded $3.9 million to Columbia University for its MySmile-Buddy program that "tests a model that uses family-level, peer-counseled, and technology-assisted behavioral risk reduction strategies…to divert children with early- and advanced-stage ECC caries from high-cost surgical dental rehabilitation to low-cost non-surgical disease management." Using the MySmileBuddy technology developed with support from the National Institute on Minority Health and Health Dis-parities, community health workers (CHWs) conduct home and community visits with parents and caregivers "to plan, implement, [facilitate] and monitor positive oral health behaviors, including dietary control and use of fluorides" with the goal of securing caries arrest and delaying and minimizing the need for reparative care. The program "was designed with a strong theoretic basis, which applies key principles of risk-based triage, early intervention, individualization, and motivational interviewing. [It] is designed to enhance parental knowledge, skills, and self-efficacy to reduce caries-related risk factors, proportionate to their child's ECC experience."[16] Parental reports of their children's oral health improvements through this program suggest that the MySmileBuddy model holds strong potential for widespread implementation as a targeted low-cost and impactful public health strategy. Half (331 of 650 parents [51%]) reported their young child's oral health to be poor (21.1%) or fair (29.8%) before the intervention whereas only 15 parents (2.3%) reported their child's oral health to be fair (2.3%) and none reported it to be poor after the intervention.

Dental public health approaches evident across these various programs include (1) a focus on populations rather than individuals; (2) attention to the highest-risk subpop-ulations; (3) engagement of preventive and disease management approaches; (4) use of evidence-based strategies; (5) involvement of nontraditional actors to deliver oral health messages; (6) coordination across care and service systems; and (7) the goal of fulfilling the triple aim by demonstrating better health outcomes at lower cost with improved patient experience.

Interest in delegations to helping professionals and lay health workers is supported by a federal regulatory change in 2014 that allows states, through a Medicaid State Plan Amendment, to determine a set of preventive services that can be delegated to nonlicensed health workers who are then paid by Medicaid. This allowance could be adopted by any state to engage CHWs in home-based and community-based oral health promotion among high-risk subpopulations by providing counseling and preventive-strategy facilitation involving fluorides.[17] The US Department of Health and Human Services Assistant Secretary for Planning and Evaluation has found that CHWs have potential "to deliver cost-effective, high-quality, and culturally-competent health services within team-based care models" and that they are most valuable when delivering "certain specific, high-value, preventive services – focused on…chronic conditions – to low-income, minority, or other underserved populations" but that "Questions remain around standardizing CHW training, certification, and licensure; establishing strong economic and other evidence to support their use; and securing reimbursement for their services to ensure financial sustainability of CHW programs."[18]

PAYMENT INNOVATION

In addition to workforce strategies, these various health care transformation initiatives explore payment methodologies that hold promise for better health outcomes at lower cost. The Health Care Payment Learning and Action Network,[19] an affinity group ol public and private health care purchasers, health care providers, employers, consumer groups, health care finance experts, and governmental agencies, in 2016 defined a rubric of alternative payment mechanisms (**Fig. 1**)[20] that feature 4 categories: category 1, fee-for-service with no linkage to quality and value; category 2, fee-for-service with linkage to quality and value through 1 of 4 levels, encompassing 2A—foundational payments for infrastructure and operations, 2B—payment for reporting, 2C—rewards for performance, and 2D—rewards and penalties based on performance; category 3, alternative payment mechanisms built on fee-for-service architecture to include level 3A—alternative payment models (APMs) with upside gainsharing and level 3B—APMs with upside gainsharing and downside risk; and category 4, population-based payment that is either 4A—condition specific or 4B—comprehensive. Each successive category provides greater opportunity for accountability and dental integration within the larger health care environment.

This succession is also reflected in **Table 1**, which relates levels of value-based reimbursement to stages of dental delivery organization and the larger health care environment. For dentistry, Tier 1 of the APM framework is most compatible with traditional fee-for-service solo and small group practices that are siloed from the larger health care delivery system. Such practices have neither the capacity nor the demand by their payers to assess the impact of their care or to become accountable to objectively measured oral health outcomes. They continue to deliver dental services with the anticipation that traditional care results in improved oral health. The Tier 2 payment approach, which retains fee-for-service but ties payment (or may even impose financial risk) to some level of accountability capacity or

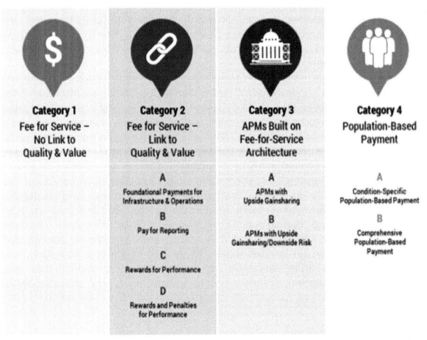

Fig. 1. APM framework (at-a-glance). (*From* Alternative Payment Model Framework and Progress Tracking Work Group. Alternative payment model (APM) framework: Final white paper. Available at: https://hcp-lan.org/workproducts/apm-whitepaper.pdf. Accessed August 4, 2017; with permission.)

Table 1
Potential dental payment and delivery trajectory

Tier	Basis for Reimbursement	Organization of Dental Delivery	Health Care Structures	Integration Characteristics
1	Fee for service (surgical focus)	Solo practitioner	Solo practice	Facilitated referrals for dental needs
2	Fee for service (prevention focus) Pay for performance to promote preventive care	Dental practice groups	Patient-centered health homes	Facilitated referrals for medical/dental needs Colocation with medical practices
3	Payment for outcomes and shared upside or downside financial risk	Regional dental networks Multi-site groups with outreach and case management	Dental ACOs	Shared financing partial integration
4	Global payments with upside and downside financial risk	Multi-site groups with outreach and case management shared with medical	Health ACOs with dental care	Fully integrated

Courtesy of Krishna Aravamudhan, BDS, MS, Chicago, IL.

performance, induces dental delivery organizations to prioritize prevention and disease management. Group dental practices or multiple dental practices networked through dental management organizations feature sufficient size and structure to develop such capacity, be paid for performance, or even accept both upside and downside financial risks. Such Tier 2 dental delivery systems can align with patient-centered medical homes that coordinate care across multiple disciplines. They may also express integration with general health care through colocation or facilitated referrals. Early efforts to institutionalize Tier 2 include pay-for-performance on specific targets, such as percentage of age-appropriate children who receive dental sealants or preventive dental visits. Tier 3 represents a transitional phase from fee-for-service to global payment with a variety of alternative payment mechanisms that enhance accountability by rewarding positive performance (upside gainsharing) or punishing failure to reach targets (downside risk). Implementation requires even larger regional dental networks with capacity for outreach and case management, large dental organizations that may function as dental accountable care organizations (ACOs). Such dental delivery systems would function best if they address a defined population and are held responsible for specified oral health targets, for example as a carve out from a larger holistic Tier 3 ACO delivery system. Transition from Tier 3 to Tier 4 is inherently disruptive and challenging because Tier 4 replaces fee-for-service payments with global payments for either a specified discipline (eg, dentistry) or for the total care of a population's people. A Tier 4 dental organization would be fully incorporated into a vertically integrated health care system like an ACO. Evident from this analysis, most dental providers practice in environments that are not amenable to APMs. The recent rapid growth, however, of very large group dental practices (those with 500 or more employees) and the accelerating aggregation of dental practices into large virtual and physical networks that share electronic health systems create new capacity to engage in advanced alternative payment mechanisms. Such large dental organizations also hold potential to

~~partner with complementary dental public health authorities in population oral health~~ management programs.

CONSTRAINTS TO NEW PAYMENT MECHANISMS AND OPPORTUNITIES FOR INNOVATION

Fig. 2 portrays critical relationships between size of health care delivery organizations (shown as small practices, independent practice associations and physician hospital organizations, and fully integrated delivery systems), type of alternative payment mechanisms (shown as fee for service, medical home payments, global case rates, and full population prepayment), and ability to assume risk and reward for health outcomes (shown as a continuum of pay for performance [P4P] opportunities, including payment for process and structure measures, payment for care coordination and short-term outcomes, and payment for health outcomes).[21] Modal dentistry today resides in the lower left corner of this representation, suggesting that it is largely unfeasible for dentists who function in small practices with fee-for-service payments to adopt performance responsibility for all but the most modest performance targets.

Beyond this organizational size constraint, Voinea-Griffin and colleagues[22] have identified several structural constraints to dentistry's adoption of value-based purchasing arrangements. These include

- Limited penetration of dentistry in public insurance and high proportion of dental expenditures that are paid out-of-pocket. There is no single payer with sufficient market leverage, except perhaps Medicaid, in pediatric dentistry to demand a change in how dentists are paid, how they are held accountable for care, or how they may assume financial upside and even downside risks.

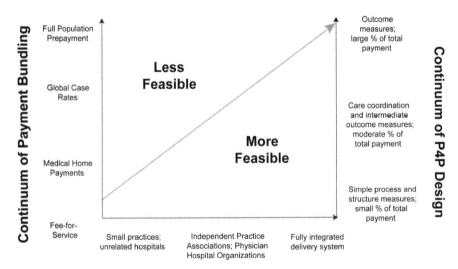

Fig. 2. Organization and payment methods. (*From* Shih A, Davis K, Schoenbaum SC, et al. Organizing the U.S. health care delivery system for high performance. Available at: http://www.commonwealthfund.org/~/media/files/publications/fund-report/2008/aug/organizing-the-u-s–health-care-delivery-system-for-high-performance/shih_organizingushltcaredeliverysys_1155-pdf.pdf. Accessed August 4, 2017; with permission.)

Only 11% of US dental spending is attributable to Medicaid and CHIP and 0.4% to Medicare and no single private payer dominates in the dental marketplace.

- Considerable variation in coverage afforded by both public insurance and private dental benefit plans. Without comparable coverage, it is difficult or impossible to compare performance across payers.
- Reluctance of the dental profession to engage in payment arrangements other than fee for service
- Lack of professional guidelines and quality measures suitable to establish performance expectations and metrics
- Considerable inter-dentist treatment variability associated with lack of evidence-based studies needed to support definitive guidelines
- Lack of valid and reliable treatment outcome measures in dentistry
- Difficulty assessing outcomes in the absence of diagnostic codes that would indicate why treatments were performed

These observers conclude, "dentistry is not ready to follow primary care [medicine] in implementing value-based purchasing programs" because too often lacking are "clear objectives, definable units of assessment, valid performance indicators, analysis and interpretation of performance data, performance standards and financial rewards."

Needed for dentistry to align itself with value-based purchasing approaches already under way in medicine is stepwise development starting with establishing administrative and clinical infrastructure, then moving to implement monitoring and evaluation processes, then to measuring clinical outcomes, and, finally, to measuring population health outcomes. Opportunities abound to do so and much work is already under way by individual dental professional organizations (in particular the American Dental Association and American Academy of Pediatric Dentistry), the Dental Quality Alliance, some insurers, and several dental management organizations. Needed infrastructure components include interoperable, networked, real-time electronic dental record platforms that allow rapid data aggregation, monitoring, and analyses (supporting big data analytics) and standardized delivery units that facilitate economies of scale, ease of maintenance and replacement, and efficiency. Processes—both administrative and clinical—similarly require standardization so that clinical activity can be readily monitored and evaluated. Clinical outcomes for dentistry are in development through the Dental Quality Alliance with the pediatric dental starter set now achieving some initial implementation. Assessing population oral health status, a core function of dental public health, which has been accomplished through epidemiologic studies, now needs to develop new capacity to measure the impact of dental care on groups' oral health status. Among processes for which dentists could be held accountable or provided bonus for achievement are

- Proportion of claims submitted electronically rather than manually
- Proportion of children who receive preventive services, including topical fluorides and sealants
- Proportion of children by risk who receive appropriate intensities of preventive and disease management interventions
- Proportion of adults with specified medical conditions (eg, diabetes) who receive appropriate periodontal care
- Proportion of treatment plan completions
- Proportion of patients treated for an emergency condition who subsequently experienced appropriate follow-up care
- Availability of after-hours emergency services[23]

Among outcomes for which dentists could be held accountable are

- Oral health maintenance evidenced as lack of caries or periodontal disease pro gression over a specified time period (monitored, for example, through service claims)
- Patient or parent self-reported oral health status
- Patient or parent self-reported oral health functionality

Overall, the evolving health care financing approaches and experiments now under way suggest that dental entrepreneurs and innovators will have a variety of opportunities to pursue greater efficiency and effectiveness. These include introducing oral health services into vertically integrated health promoting systems that are funded through global payment; expanding the concept of dental care to include attention to social and behavioral determinants of health in the contexts of life span and common determinants with other chronic health conditions,[24] engaging nontraditional providers,[25] distinguishing delivery systems by performance, and integrating public health and clinical approaches to effectuate true population health management.[26]

TRENDS IN US DENTAL CARE FINANCING

In aggregate at the total population level, US dental care today is financed substantially by private insurance (47%), out-of-pocket personal expenditures (40%), and public insurance (12%) with the remaining 2% attributable to direct care programs like the Indian Health Service, Department of Veterans Affairs, and Department of Defense (**Fig. 3**). Historically, there has been a long-term increase in dental care financed by private insurance (from 2% to 47% between 1960 and 2015) and public insurance (from 0% to 12%) and a commensurate decline in out-of-pocket expenditures (from 96% to 40%).

Not evident from these aggregate findings is a significant difference in dental care financing by population age. For US adults, private dental insurance has been in modest decline since peaking in 1996 at 52% whereas public insurance remains spotty because of variations in adult dental Medicaid coverage by state. For US children—half of whom have public insurance (Medicaid and CHIP)—the contribution of Medicaid and CHIP is significantly greater whereas out-of-pocket expenditures are

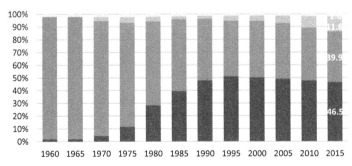

Fig. 3. Dental care financing 1960 to 2015, by source. (*Data from* Centers for Medicare & Medicaid Services. National health expenditure data. Available at: https://www.cms.gov/ Research-Statistics-Data-and-Systems/Statistics-Trends-and-Reports/NationalHealthExpendData/ NationalHealthAccountsHistorical.html. Accessed August 4, 2017.)

lesser. With no substantive dental benefit in Medicare, older adults pay disproportionately out-of-pocket for dental care.

The ACA, like the Medicaid Early and Periodic Screening, Diagnostic, and Treatment (EPSDT) pediatric benefit in 1967 and CHIP Reauthorization in 2010, established a guaranteed dental insurance benefit for children but not for adults. Through the combination of Medicaid EPSDT, CHIP, and the ACA EHBs that apply to private coverage, almost all child citizens have a path to dental coverage that is robust and comprehensive, inclusive of prevention, restoration, and orthodontic care.

On becoming the majority party in the US Congress and holding the Presidency as of January 2017, Republican policymakers have revisited core elements of the ACA with the goal of aligning US health care financing with conservative political ideologies and markedly reducing the financial contribution of the federal government to Medicaid. The Tax Cuts and Jobs Act, enacted in December 2017, eliminated the individual mandate that requires everyone to obtain and maintain health insurance to prevent adverse selection and the resultant insurance death spiral. Other legislative proposals call for greater roles for state-level policymaking, including determination of benefits, thereby excluding some benefits that are considered "essential" under the ACA; increased responsibility of states for managing the financing of health care in the name of federalism with a concomitant reduction in the federal government's financial contributions by means of block grants and per capita caps; a smaller role for governments at all levels in incentivizing or punishing provider behaviors; and a larger role for the marketplace to address challenges in health care financing.

Initial repeal-and-replace legislation passed by the House of Representatives in May 2017, the American Health Care Act, and by the US Senate in June 2017, the Better Care Reconciliation Act, incorporated these policy shifts. According to scoring by the nonpartisan Congressional Budget Office, this House bill would have generate $119 billion in federal health care savings over 10 years while causing 23 million people to lose health coverage[27] whereas the Senate bill would have generate $321 billion in potential deficit reduction over 10 years while causing 22 million people to lose health coverage.[28] Specific to pediatric oral health services, the report on the House bill notes, "Services or benefits likely to be excluded from the EHBs in some states include maternity care, mental health and substance abuse benefits, rehabilitative and habilitative services, and pediatric dental benefits." The legislation would additionally have lifted the ban on annual and lifetime limits on any covered benefits that are no longer deemed essential by a state.

After the US Senate Republican majority's narrow failure to pass partisan "repeal and replace," "repeal and delay," and "skinny repeal" bills in July 2017, the ACA remains in place. As of August 2017, multiple bipartisan efforts were in development to stabilize insurance markets and retain high levels of coverage. President Trump, however, continued to caution that "Obamacare will implode" and may facilitate such failure by not enforcing the individual mandate requirement, not promoting enrollment through advertising and outreach, imposing a work requirement on Medicaid recipients, and reducing the federal portion of premium, copay, and deductible payments for modest-income enrollees.[29] Whatever policy remedies the Congress may next implement to address shortcomings of the ACA will confront the same tradeoffs and challenges that existed before passage of the ACA in 2010. The US will continue to confront per capita health care costs that are considerably higher than in comparable developed countries while producing lesser health outcomes,[30] continue to deal with medical inflation that exceeds overall inflation, continue to seek politically acceptable approaches to encouraging or requiring coverage and stabilizing the health insurance marketplace, address those who last insurances, ensure meaningful benefits, and control costs. As President Trump acknowledged when addressing the nation's governors on February 28, 2017, health care "is an unbelievably complex subject," adding "nobody knew health care could be so complicated." As a sector of the US economy that consumes 17% of gross domestic product, employs 1 in 10 employed persons in the United States, consumes significant federal dollars, and has an impact every person in the United States, health care requires sophisticated policymaking that seeks to maximize outcomes while causing the least possible harm.

IMPLICATIONS FOR DENTAL PUBLIC HEALTH

Public health, by definition, concerns itself with the health and welfare of everyone. It builds on a holistic view of health that includes attention to the full range of biological, social, environmental, and behavioral determinants. Therefore, it is natural to public health to seek improvements in health by addressing income, employment, housing, and food insecurities as well as by providing direct health services. In contrast, a majority of US health care delivery and financing systems are narrowly focused and primarily privately managed by employers and their contractors. Private systems are concerned with the particular subpopulation covered by a particular private insurance program and served by a particular group of participating providers. By default, the public health sector has largely assumed responsibility for those who fall outside these employer-based private systems—socially vulnerable children and aged, the poor, and the disabled. Public health is, therefore, often conflated with the health care safety net, which includes public insurance (primarily Medicaid) and a network of federally qualified and similar health centers. It receives lesser attention for its other core responsibilities—promoting prevention, educating the public, managing societal and environmental risks, implementing policy, and monitoring health status of populations.

This private-public dichotomy is being conceptually challenged by the advent of value-based approaches to health management and purchasing. Convergence is emerging as private systems recognize that the "value" they seek—better health outcomes at lower cost—can be attained in large part through attention to public health approaches that include health prevention, education, risk management, and disease management and that population-level monitoring is essential to measure outcomes. This convergence supports the advent of health systems that approach health holistically to replace health care systems that focus disproportionately on medical and surgical interventions to address extant disease. Nascent ACOs and patient-centered medical homes are actively experimenting with this transformation for medical care but have attended little to dental reform.

Looking to the future, dental public health as a specialty can be expected to gain ever-greater relevance and deliver ever-greater impact as it contributes its perspectives, tools, and talents to evolving US health and health-financing systems.

REFERENCES

1. Available at: www.investopedia.com/terms/v/valueproposition.asp. Accessed August 4, 2017.
2. Kissick W. Medicine's Dilemmas: infinite needs versus finite resources. New Haven (CT): Yale University Press; 1994.
3. Institute for Healthcare Improvement. IHI triple aim initiative: better care for individuals, better health for populations, and lower per capita costs. Available at: http://www.ihi.org/Engage/Initiatives/TripleAim/Pages/default.aspx. Accessed May 27, 2017.

4. Centers for Medicare and Medicaid Services. CMS' value-based programs. Available at: https://www.cms.gov/Medicare/Quality-Initiatives-Patient-Assessment-Instruments/Value-Based-Programs/Value-Based-Programs.html. Accessed May 27, 2017.

5. Centers for Medicare and Medicaid Services. Health care innovation. Our mission. Available at: https://innovation.cms.gov/about/Our-Mission/index.html. Accessed May 28, 2017.

6. Gates A. Rudowitz R, Guyer J. An overview of delivery system reform incentive payment waivers. Henry J. Kaiser Family Foundation. 2014. Available at: http://kff.org/medicaid/issue-brief/an-overview-of-delivery-system-reform-incentive-payment-waivers/. Accessed May 27, 2017.

7. Centers for Medicare and Medicaid Services. Health Care Innovation Awards. Available at: https://innovation.cms.gov/initiatives/Health-Care-Innovation-Awards. Accessed May 27, 2017.

8. Bodenheimer T, Wagner EH, Grumbach K. Improving Primary care for Patients with Chronic Illness. J Am Med Assoc 2002;228(14):1775–9.

9. Brino A. MACPAC report on Medicaid touts DSRIP, warns about behavioral and dental health. Portland (ME): HealthCareFinance; 2015. Available at: http://www.healthcarefinancenews.com/news/macpac-report-medicaid-touts-dsrip-warns-about-behavioral-and-dental-health. Accessed May 27, 2017.

10. New York State Department of Health. DSRIP domain 4 and the prevention agenda. Available at: https://www.health.ny.gov/health_care/medicaid/redesign/dsrip/2016/d4guidance_2015-06-08_final.htm. Accessed May 27, 2017.

11. Chazin S, Crawford M. Oral health integration in statewide delivery system and payment reform. Trenton (NJ): Center for Heatlh Care Strategies, Inc; 2016. Available at: http://www.chcs.org/media/Oral-Health-Integration-Opportunities-Brief-052516-FINAL.pdf. Accessed May 27, 2017.

12. Centers for Medicare and Medicaid Services, Center for Medicaid and CHIP Services, Medicaid Innovation Accelerator Program/CMS Oral Health Initiative. Children's Oral Health Initiative Value-Based Payment Technical Support Program Overview. 2017. Available at: https://www.medicaid.gov/state-resource-center/innovation-accelerator-program/iap-downloads/functional-areas/ohi-program-overview.pdf. Accessed May 27, 2017.

13. Centers for Medicare and Medicaid Services: Center for Medicare and Medicaid Innovation, Budget Overview. Available at: https://www.hhs.gov/about/budget/fy2015/budget-in-brief/cms/innovation-programs/index.html. Accessed August 4, 2017.

14. Center for Medicare and Medicaid Services. Health care innovation awards round one project profiles. Delta Dental Plan of South Dakota. Available at: https://innovation.cms.gov/files/x/hcia-project-profiles.pdf. Accessed May 28, 2017.

15. Center for Medicare and Medicaid Services. Health Care Innovation Awards Round Two: Michigan – Altarum Institute. Available at: https://innovation.cms.gov/initiatives/Health-Care-Innovation-Awards-Round-Two/Michigan.html. Accessed May 28, 2017.

16. Center for Medicare and Medicaid Services. Health Care Innovation Awards Round Two: New York – Trustees of Columbia University in the City of New York. Available at: https://innovation.cms.gov/initiatives/Health-Care-Innovation-Awards-Round-Two/New-York.html. Accessed May 28, 2017.

17. Update on Preventive Services Initiatives. CMCS Informational Bulletin. 11/27/13. Available at: https://www.medicaid.gov/Federal-Policy-Guidance/Downloads/CIB-11-27-2013-Prevention.pdf. Accessed January 28, 2016.

18. Snyder JL. Community health workers: roles and opportunities in health care delivery system reform. Department of Health and Human Services. Washington DC: ASPE Issue Brief; 2016. Available at: https://aspe.hhs.gov/system/files/pdf/168956/CHWPolicy.pdf. Accessed May 28, 2017.

19. HCP-LAN (Health Care Payment Learning & Action Network). Webpage Available at: https://hcp-lan.org/. Accessed May 28, 2017.

20. HCP-LAN. Alternative Payment Model Framework and Progress Tracking Work Group. Alternative Payment Model (APM) Framework: A White Paper. 2016. Available at: https://hcp-lan.org/workproducts/apm-whitepaper.pdf. Accessed May 28, 2017.

21. Shih A, Davis K, Schoenbaum SC, et al. Organizing the US healthcare delivery system for high performance. New York: The Commonwealth Fund Commission on a High Performance Health System; 2008. Available at: http://www.commonwealthfund.org/~/media/files/publications/fund-report/2008/aug/organizing-the-u-s–health-care-delivery-system-for-high-performance/shih_organizingushltcaredeliverysys_1155-pdf.pdf. Accessed May 28, 2017.

22. Voinea-Griffin A, Fellows JL, Rindal DB, et al. Pay for performance: will dentistry follow? BMC Oral Health 2010;10:9. Available at: www.biomedcentral.com/1472-6831/10/9.

23. Oregon Health Authority. Oral Health in Oregon's CCOs: a Metrics Report. 2017. Available at: https://www.oregon.gov/oha/analytics/Documents/oral-health-ccos.pdf. Accessed June 3, 2017.

24. da Foncesca M, Avenetti F. Social determinants of pediatric oral health. Dent Clin North Am 2017;64(3):519–32.

25. Edelstein BL. Improving pediatric oral health through interprofessional interventions. Dent Clin North Am 2017;63(3):589–606.

26. Rubin MS, Edelstein BL. Perspectives on evolving dental care payment and delivery models. J Am Dent Assoc 2016;147:50–6.

27. Congressional Budget Office. Cost estimate HR1628 American Health Care Act passed by the House of Representatives on May 4, 2017. 2017. Available at: https://www.cbo.gov/system/files/115th-congress-2017-2018/costestimate/hr1628aspassed.pdf. Accessed June 5, 2017.

28. Available at: https://www.cbo.gov/system/files/115th-congress-2017-2018/costestimate/52849-hr1628senate.pdf. Accessed August 4, 2017.

29. Park H, Sanger-Katz M. Three things trump is already doing to 'Let Obamacare Implode'. New York Times 2017. Available at: https://www.nytimes.com/interactive/2017/07/19/us/what-trump-can-do-to-let-obamacare-fail.html.

30. Schneider EC, Sarnak DO, Sqauires D, et al. Mirror, Mirror 2017: International Comparison Reflects Flaws and Opportunities for Better U.S. Health Care. Interactive website. Available at: http://www.commonwealthfund.org/interactives/2017/july/mirror-mirror/. Accessed August 4, 2017.

Moving?

Make sure your subscription moves with you!

To notify us of your new address, find your **Clinics Account Number** (located on your mailing label above your name), and contact customer service at:

Email: journalscustomerservice-usa@elsevier.com

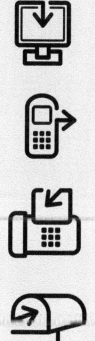

800-654-2452 (subscribers in the U.S. & Canada)
314-447-8871 (subscribers outside of the U.S. & Canada)

Fax number: 314-447-8029

Elsevier Health Sciences Division
Subscription Customer Service
3251 Riverport Lane
Maryland Heights, MO 63043

*To ensure uninterrupted delivery of your subscription, please notify us at least 4 weeks in advance of move.

Printed and bound by CPI Group (UK) Ltd, Croydon, CR0 4YY

03/10/2024

01040395-0020